Neuroevolutional Approach to Cerebral Palsy and Speech

EDWARD D. MYSAK, Ph.D.

Professor of Speech Pathology
Chairman, Department of Speech Pathology and Audiology
Director, Speech and Hearing Center
Teachers College, Columbia University
Fellow of the American Speech and Hearing Association

TEACHERS COLLEGE PRESS

Teachers College, Columbia University
New York, New York

*To all those children
who may benefit in some way
from the ideas
expressed in this book*

Preface to the New Edition

In the preface of the first edition of this book, which was entitled, *Principles of a Reflex Therapy Approach to Cerebral Palsy*, the author stated that since many present-day conventional treatments of cerebral palsy were not as effective as would be desired, cerebral palsy specialists should consider it a responsibility to thoroughly investigate any new approaches which might prove of some value. In that spirit, the stated purpose of the first edition was to discuss the important contributions that a neurophysiologically-oriented approach might make to the habilitation of the child with cerebral palsy.

Now about four years later, the author is pleased to report that he senses from the literature, and from his contacts with various professionals involved in the area of cerebral palsy habilitation, a steady increase in the application of neurophysiological concepts in treatment programs for the cerebral palsied.

In this new edition, the author has endeavored to update the material in light of the fast-growing literature in the area and as a result of his continued experimentation with neurotherapy techniques. The revision of the book's title is intended to reflect some further development in the author's thinking which, hopefully, will be brought out in the body of the book. Other additions include illustrations in the chapter on the evolution of the human CNS, a much expanded speech section, and the inclusion of an index.

In the preface of the first edition, the author also acknowledged the substantial extent which the material he presented was based on the ideas and writings of Dr. and Mrs. Karel Bobath, and on the concepts of the late and renowned Dr. Hughlings Jackson. He also extended his sincere appreciation to the staff of the Newington Hospital for Crippled Children in Newington, Connecticut, where the author first applied the principles and methods of a neurologically-oriented treatment approach to cerebral palsy. The author wishes to reiterate his indebtedness to all these people for their continuing and important influences on this revised edition.

Finally, the author wishes to extend his sincere appreciation to all those individuals who helped to prepare this book. Specifically, he wishes to express his thanks to Theresa M. Mysak for her patient ear and patient proofreading, and to Mrs. Mary Katanik for her excellent typing of the original manuscript.

E.D.M.

Contents

PART ONE

Principles and Rationale
of Neurotherapy

CHAPTER ONE

Background Theory

As an introduction here the author has decided to restate and to embellish certain ideas which he used as introductory material in a chapter found in the proceedings of a workshop on speech and language therapy with the cerebral palsied child (Mysak, 1964).

There it was stated that at least three approaches to the management of human disorders may be recognized: the symptomatic, the etiologic, and the prophylactic. During the course of any one particular treatment history various combinations of these three approaches may be utilized. However, whichever approach or combinations of approaches are being employed at any one time is usually related to (1) the amount of available knowledge with respect to the particular disease process; (2) the available treatment methods and techniques; and (3) the number of trained specialists available to employ the treatment methods and techniques. This means that whenever a disease and its cause are well understood there is a good chance that the highest form of management, the prophylactic or preventive type, might eventually become possible. As an example, the discovery and analysis of polio viruses was followed by the development of vaccines which resulted in preventive medicine against poliomyelitis. Before the vaccine was discovered, however, the treatment for polio was basically symptomatic, which meant there was first an attempt to relieve the fever and then, after the disease ran its course, braces and physical therapy were usually prescribed for one of its frequent symptoms, paraplegia. However, this approach to polio was usually of little value in relieving, to any substantial degree, the symptoms of paraplegia.

A similar type of management history may be described for that form of cerebral palsy resulting from incompatible bloods (Rh factor) between a mother and her infant. Before this particular disease process was well understood, certain mothers would give birth to infants who, within twenty-four hours or so, showed symptoms of jaundice and who

3

later on may have shown symptoms of athetosis and auditory disorder. Once the problem was manifested, the child was, for the most part, treated symptomatically; that is, he may have received special orthopedic devices for the musculoskeletal symptoms of his neurophysiological disorder, plus conventional training for developing the best use of his disordered motor patterns. As more was learned about this disease, an etiologic form of management evolved which involved the massive replacement of the affected blood of the child at birth with normal blood. When this treatment is thoroughly successful, it may be described as representing a causal prophylactic form of management.

Prophylaxis proper with respect to Rh athetosis is based on (1) the education of health professionals and the general public concerning the possible consequences of Rh negative mothers conceiving second and third Rh positive children; and (2) the eventual development of the means of inhibiting the build-up of specific antibodies within pregnant Rh negative females. (It is the understanding of the author that such means are presently under investigation.)

It would be good indeed if the causes of other forms of cerebral palsy were understood equally as well and if more of them could be managed by etiologic and prophylactic means. But, alas, this is not the situation. The majority of the cerebral palsies are still primarily treated via symptomatic approaches. This usually means that little direct attention is paid to the primary neurophysiological disturbance shown by these children, but when they develop secondary muscle, tendon, and bone anomalies, these are the problems which are basically treated. More specifically, conventional approaches to the habilitation of the cerebral palsied have, for the most part, been represented by treatment techniques having musculoskeletal orientations. Such therapy programs usually include direct teaching of motor tasks plus the use of special devices and various orthopedic surgical procedures. However, because symptomatically-oriented treatments are often so frustrating and minimally effective, an ever-increasing number of specialists are seeking for more effective, neurophysiologically-based approaches to the problem. For example, there have been reports in the literature of attempts at employing special types of neurosurgery (e.g., Myers, 1956) as well as numerous attempts in the use of various drug therapies (e.g., Mautner, 1956). Unfortunately, these treatment approaches have shown only limited results. It is hoped that with more research and work such etiologically-oriented managements will bring greater results, and eventually that additional prophylactic measures will also be developed. With respect to causal prophylactic approaches to cerebral palsy, the developing speciality of fetology which includes the study and practice of intrauterine treatment of fetuses, and the recent report

of the use of decompression techniques (Heyns, 1962) during pregnancy and delivery periods certainly appear interesting and promising.

While research is continuing in the use of neurosurgery and drugs,
and in prophylaxis of cerebral palsy, it is clear that cerebral palsy
specialists should be encouraged to explore and develop etiologically-
oriented speech, occupational, and physical therapies. One such approach, which involves the application of neurophysiological theory to
the problem, was introduced by the Bobaths and has shown encouraging results. The Bobaths have described their theories in numerous
articles. (See for example, Bobath, B., 1955, 1963; Bobath, K., 1959;
and Bobath and Bobath, 1964.) The material presented in this book is
derived for the most part from experiences in the study and application of their basic therapy principles, as well as from the study of the
neurophysiological therapy concepts of Fay (1948), Kabat (1952), and
Rood (1954) over a period of about nine years. In the course of this
study and application by the author, there has been a continuing development in principles, rationale, and techniques of treatment as reflected in the following publications: three films (Mysak, 1958, 1960,
1962); three journal articles (Mysak, 1959, 1963, and Mysak and
Fiorentino, 1961); a chapter (Mysak, 1965); and the first edition of
this book published in 1963.

The specific purposes of this second edition are: (1) To present as
clearly and as concisely as possible theoretical information on a neurophysiologically-based approach to cerebral palsy habilitation. The
term neuroevolutional, found in the title of this new edition, is used to
indicate that the therapy approach will draw extensively from information pertaining to human, neurological ontogenesis. (2) To describe
the application of neuroevolutional concepts to cerebral palsy habilitation in general. (3) To describe in detail the application of neuroevolutional concepts to oropharyngeal maturation, to cerebral palsy
respiratory-phonatory-articulatory disorders, and to therapy procedures for these disorders.

JACKSONIAN OBSERVATIONS ON NEUROPATHOLOGY

In order to understand better neurotherapy concepts as they pertain
to cerebral palsy, it is important that the reader become acquainted
with certain theories and observations on neuropathology as expressed
by Jackson (1958).

Support for a neurotherapy orientation to cerebral palsy may be
drawn from Jackson's concepts of the evolution and dissolution of the
nervous system, and duplex symptomatology in nervous diseases.

Evolution and Dissolution of the Nervous System

Jackson described evolution as "an ascending development in a particular order" (Jackson, 1958, p. 46). The progression is from CNS centers which are relatively well organized at birth, or the lowest centers: to those which are continually organizing through life, or the highest centers. A progression from the most simple to the most complex; from the most automatic to the least automatic. According to Jackson (1958, p. 46), dissolution, or the "reverse of the process of evolution," is the reduction of CNS activity from least organized, most complex, and least automatic toward the most organized, most simple, and most automatic. In other words, in a case of neuropathology, dissolution represents reduction to a lower level of neurophysiological ontogenesis. Further, Jackson spoke of uniform and local dissolutions and also depths of dissolution. By uniform dissolution, he meant that the whole nervous system was relatively evenly reversed, while by local dissolution, he meant that disease of a part of the nervous system caused a local reversal of evolution.

> Disease may occur on any evolutionary level, on one side or on both sides; it may affect the sensory elements chiefly, or the motor elements chiefly (1958, p. 47).

In terms of depth of dissolution, Jackson stated:

> An injurious agency, such as alcohol, taken into the system, flows to all parts of it; but the highest centres, being least organized, "give out" first and most; the middle centres, being more organized, resist longer; and the lowest centres, being most organized, resist longest (1958, p. 47).

Duplex Symptomatology

Jackson believed that the symptomatology of all nervous diseases is duplex, or characterized by both a positive and a negative element. He described negative symptoms as reflecting loss or defect of function and positive symptoms as reflecting involuntary activities. According to Jackson, destructive lesions produce loss or defect of function, or negative symptoms; they could never be responsible for positive symptoms. Involuntary activities or positive symptoms are the result of the released activity of lower brain centers due to the removal of some inhibitory mechanism by the negative lesion. In terms of the doctrine of dissolution, the negative element is loss of the least organized, most complex, and least automatic functioning; the positive element is the release of more organized, less complex, and more automatic functioning.

Jackson presented various examples (1958, pp. 48, 49) which may serve to illustrate the concept of duplex symptomatology. In speaking of hemiplegia, "owing to destruction of part of a plexus in the mid-region of the brain," he said there is

> loss of more or fewer of the most voluntary movements of one side of the body; we find that the arm, the more voluntary limb, suffers the more and the longer; we find, too, that the most voluntary part of the face suffers more than the rest of the face.

With respect to the positive and negative elements, Jackson states that

> although the unilateral movements (the more voluntary) are lost, the more automatic, the bilateral, are retained.

As one example of duplex symptomatology at the highest center, Jackson described "delirium in acute non-cerebral disease."

> The patient's condition is partly negative and partly positive. Negatively, he ceases to know that he is in hospital, and ceases to recognize persons about him . . . he is defectively conscious . . . We may conveniently say that it shows loss of function of the topmost "layer" of his highest centres . . . The other half of his condition is positive. Besides his not knowings, there are his wrong knowings. He imagines himself to be at home or at work, and acts, as far as practicable, as if he were.

With these Jacksonian concepts in mind, it is proposed that cerebral palsy may also be viewed in terms of the doctrine of evolution and dissolution of the CNS and in terms of duplex symptomatology.

In cerebral palsy we find children who may be limited to such infantile positions as supine or sitting (negative symptoms of arrested or retarded neuromotor development) and who also show the appropriate background infantile reflexes (positive symptoms). That is, a particular child may be showing the general reflexes found in the infant of six months or less and, accordingly, he reflects the associated motor activity. (See Appendix A.) Along these lines, Twitchell (1965), in discussing certain children whose motor development is stretched out over a five- or six-year period, stated, ". . . In a sense, the patient with cerebral palsy represents a still more profound physiological defect in sensory-motor maturation or integration with a hypertrophy of various infantile reflexes."

CEREBRAL PALSY AS A REFLECTION OF
DISTURBED NEURO-ONTOGENESIS

Applying Jackson's concepts of evolution and dissolution of the nervous system and duplex symptomatology in neuropathologies to the condition of cerebral palsy, a given case of cerebral palsy may be viewed as reflecting: (1) nervous system dissolution, in cases of acquired cerebral palsy where a normal child is neurophysiologically reduced as a result of some brain disease; or, (2) nervous system arrestment or retardation, in cases of congenital cerebral palsy. In both cases, positive and negative symptoms are manifested.

Negative symptoms, or loss or defect of function symptoms, are related to involvement of the least organized, most complex and least automatic centers of the central nervous system (e.g., sensorimotor integration centers which subserve * righting and equilibrium reactions). While the positive symptoms, or involuntary activity symptoms, are related to release of the more organized, less complex, and more automatic centers of the central nervous system (e.g., sensorimotor integration centers which subserve spinal and brain stem reflexes).

This definition differs from the one presented by the author in an article (Mysak, 1959) describing the Bobath orientation to the problem. Further study and application of Jacksonian concepts of neuropathology resulted in the formulation of the revised description.

With this interesting orientation to the understanding of the child with cerebral palsy, questions concerning possible neurophysiologically-based treatment techniques are easily generated. For example, is it possible to stimulate in some manner further evolution or re-evolution of the central nervous system? Is it possible that retained or released positive symptoms are reflections of a lower-center domination over a system which has greater potential for CNS maturation or function? Is it possible to shunt afferent inflow beyond lower-order sensorimotor integration centers so that higher-order sensorimotor integration may take place?

Proposed answers to these and other questions will be found in those sections and chapters of the book devoted to neurotherapy procedures. However, because the definition, assessment, and treatment of cerebral palsy in this book are based on concepts of human, neuro-ontogenesis and neuro-phylo-ontogenesis, and because many specialists are not adequately familiar with these concepts, the chapters devoted to treatment will be preceded by one designed to provide the reader with necessary information on these subjects.

In the way of clarifying the word "neuro-phylo-ontogenesis," it is a term which describes the "recapitulation theory" as it pertains to the evolution of the nervous system. In turn, the term recapitulation refers to the repetition in ontogeny of the evolutionary stages through which the species evolved.

---

* The nature and purpose of the equilibrium and righting reactions and the brain stem and spinal reflexes will be discussed·in Chapter Two.

Travis (1931, p. 15) stated, "It is believed that each cardinal evolutionary step in nervous development is recorded as a more or less distinct level in the human nervous equipment . . ." Travis (1931, p. 22) goes on to indicate that higher centers assume a directive and regulatory control over the lower centers which continue to serve their basic functions. Other selected and related comments include: ". . . in the development of neuromotor activity, ontogeny may recapitulate phylogeny just as it does in the development of the pharynx . . ." (Swinyard, 1967, p. 219); ". . . there appears to be in the behavior repertoire of the newborn infant certain patterns which reflect a phyletic heritage" (McGraw, 1962, p. 11); and, finally, "During the first years of life the infant passes through the stage of the quadruped and thus repeats the phylogenetic pattern of man" (Peiper, 1963, p. 177).

REFERENCES

Bobath, B. "The treatment of motor disorders of pyramidal and extrapyramidal origin by reflex inhibition and by facilitation of movements," *Physiotherapy*, 41 (1955), 146–153.

Bobath, B. "Treatment principles and planning in cerebral palsy," *Physiotherapy* (April, 1963), 1–3.

Bobath, K. "The neuropathology of cerebral palsy and its importance in treatment and diagnosis," *Cerebral Palsy Bull.* (Winter, 1959), 13–33.

Bobath, K. and Bobath, B. "The facilitation of normal postural reactions and movements in the treatment of cerebral palsy," *Physiotherapy* (August, 1964), 3–19.

Fay, T. "Neurophysical aspects of therapy in cerebral palsy," *Arch. Phys. Med.*, 29 (1948), 327–334.

Heyns, O. S. "Use of abdominal decompression in pregnancy and labour to improve foetal oxygenation," *Develop. Med. Child Neurol.*, 4 (1962), 473–482.

Jackson, J. H. "Evolution and Dissolution of the Nervous System" in James Taylor (Ed.), *Selected Writings of John Hughlings Jackson*, Vol. 2, New York: Basic Books, Inc., 1958.

Kabat, H. "Central facilitation; the basis of treatment for paralysis," *Permanente Foundation Med. Bull.*, 10 (1952), 190–204.

Mautner, H. "Drug therapy in cerebral palsy," *Arch. Pediat.*, 73 (1956), 351–381.

McGraw, Myrtle B. *The Neuromuscular Maturation of the Human Infant.* New York: Hafner Publishing Co., 1962.

Myers, R. "Results of bilateral intermediate midbrain crusotomy in seven cases of severe athetotic and dystonic quadriparesis," *Amer. J. Phys. Med.*, 35 (1956), 84–105.

Mysak, E. D. The Bobath Approach to Cerebral Palsy Habilitation. Film released by the Newington Hospital for Crippled Children, Newington, Connecticut, July, 1958.

Mysak, E. D. "Significance of neurophysiological orientation to cerebral palsy habilitation," *J. Speech Hearing Dis.*, 24 (1959), 221–230.

Mysak, E. D. Pilot Study Films of a Neurophysiological Approach to Cerebral Palsy Habilitation. Film released by the Newington Hospital for Crippled Children, Newington, Connecticut, June, 1960.

Mysak, E. D. Pilot Study Films of a Neurophysiological Approach to Cerebral Palsy Habilitation: Part Two. Film released by the Newington Hospital for Crippled Children, Newington, Connecticut, November, 1962.

Mysak, E. D. "Dysarthria and oropharyngeal reflexology: a review," *J. Speech Hearing Dis.*, 28 (1963), 252–260.

Mysak, E. D. "Reflex Therapy and Cerebral Palsy Habilitation" in W. T. Daley (Ed.), *Speech and Language Therapy with the Cerebral Palsied Child.* Washington, D.C.: The Catholic University of America Press, 1965.

Mysak, E. D. and Fiorentino, M. R. "Neurophysiological considerations in occupational therapy for the cerebral palsied," *Amer. J. Occup. Ther.*, 15 (1961), 112–117.

Peiper, A. *Cerebral Function in Infancy and Childhood.* New York: Consultants Bureau, 1963.

Rood, M. "Neurophysiological reactions as a basis for physical therapy," *Phys. Therapy Rev.*, 34 (1954), 444–449.

Swinyard, C. A. "Developmental aspects of neurological structure relevant to cerebral palsy," *Develop. Med. Child Neurol.*, 9 (1967), 216–221.

Travis, L. E. *Speech Pathology.* New York: D. Appleton Century Co., 1931.

Twitchell, T. E. "Variations and abnormalities of motor development," *J. Amer. Phys. Ther. Assoc.*, 45 (1965), 424–430.

CHAPTER TWO

Human Neuroevolution

A review of normal human neuroevolution should serve at least two purposes. First, it should help clarify Jackson's concept of an ascending development of brain center control in the normal individual. Second, with respect to the cerebral palsied individual, it should aid clinicians in evaluating the child's level of nervous system arrestment, retardation, or dissolution; it should enable the clinician to identify the undesirable retained or released positive symptoms; and it should allow the clinician to determine which righting and equilibrium reactions should be stimulated or re-stimulated in order to improve the child's over-all sensorimotor integration status.

The description of human neuroevolution will proceed from the lowest infantile levels to the highest mature levels.

SPINAL REFLEXES

Prior to describing the spinal reflexes, it would be well to acquaint the reader with certain testing considerations, especially if he intends to utilize the information presented to test the cerebral palsied. The tester, of course, should first apply the adequate stimulus in the recommended position and observe whether or not the expected movement, sequence of movements, and(or) posture has occurred. If the expected response does not occur however, he should also observe and attempt the following: (1) observe whether the stimulus has at least caused appropriate changes in muscle tone, if not actual movements and postural changes, (2) apply the stimulus against resistance, and (3) where appropriate, apply the stimulus in different positions and situations, for example, during sitting, standing and while walking. In short, when evaluating the cerebral palsied, the tester should make every effort to collect all information that may be of value in diagnosis and in planning a treatment program.

11

Testing for the presence of the asymmetrical tonic neck reflex may be used as a specific example of a somewhat unusual testing situation. It may be found that lateralizing the head with the child in supine does not elicit the expected flexion of the skull limbs and extension of the face limbs. However, if the child is asked to right his lateralized head while the tester resists the movement, the expected response may now be observed to occur, or at least the appropriate muscle tone may appear in the limbs. In one instance, signs of the asymmetrical tonic neck reflex appeared only when the child's head was lateralized during his attempts to walk.

Returning to the discussion of spinal reflexes, these reflexes are mediated by areas of the CNS up to the base of the fourth ventricle; they are "phasic" or movement reflexes and they coordinate the muscles of the limbs in patterns of either total flexion or extension. They were studied by Sherrington (1939) in laboratory experiments on cats. These reflexes may or may not be elicited in normal infants up to two months of age. Positive reactions beyond two months of age may be an indication of CNS dysmaturation.

Flexor Withdrawal

With the leg in an extended position, stimulation of the sole of the foot (usually by pricking) produces extension of the toes, dorsiflexion of the foot, and flexion of the leg and thigh, or the flexor withdrawal reflex. To elicit: place the individual in a supine position and stimulate the sole of the foot. A positive reaction is characterized by generalized flexion of the extended, stimulated limb.

Extensor Thrust

With the leg in a flexed position, stimulation of the sole of the foot produces extension at all joints by contraction of all extensor muscles and inhibition of the flexor muscles, or the extensor thrust reflex. To elicit: place the individual in a supine position and stimulate the flexed limb as described.

Crossed Extension

In the crossed extension reflex, flexion of one limb elicits extension of all joints of the contralateral flexed limb. To elicit: place the individual in a supine position and flex one leg; upon leg flexion, the other flexed leg extends. Or maintain one leg in extension and rub the sole of the foot of this leg; a positive response in the opposite limb is one of flexion and then extension and adduction, internal rotation, and extension and fanning of the toes.

Figure 1 shows how the three spinal reflexes are elicited as well as the sequence of movements involved.

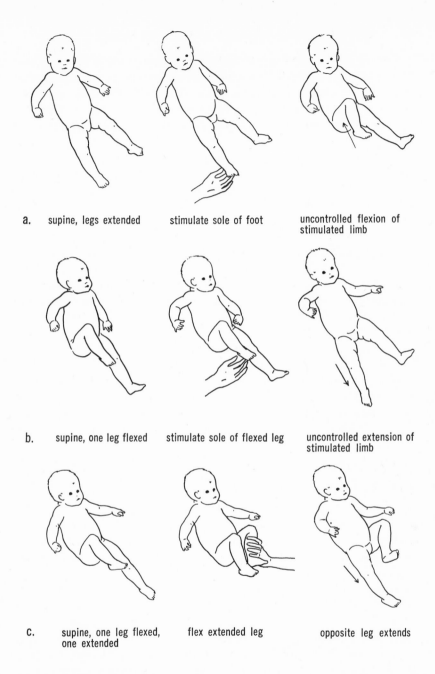

a.   supine, legs extended   stimulate sole of foot   uncontrolled flexion of
                                                                               stimulated limb

b.   supine, one leg flexed   stimulate sole of flexed leg   uncontrolled extension of
                                                                               stimulated limb

c.   supine, one leg flexed,   flex extended leg   opposite leg extends
    one extended

Figure 1. Spinal reflexes: elicitation and characteristic movements.
a. flexor withdrawal. b. extensor thrust. c. crossed extension.

BRAIN STEM REFLEXES

Brain stem reflexes are mediated by areas from the eighth nerve nucleus to below the red nucleus. They are "static" postural reflexes and effect changes in the distribution of muscle tone throughout the body. They may be activated when there is a change in the position of the head and body in space (stimulation of the labyrinths), or when there is a change in the position of the head in relation to the body (stimulation of the proprioceptors of the neck). They were studied in laboratory animals by Sherrington (1939, 1947) and Magnus (1926). These reflexes may or may not be elicited in the normal child within the first four to six months. Persistence of these reflexes beyond six months may be an indication of CNS dysmaturation.

Asymmetrical Tonic Neck Reflex

The asymmetrical tonic neck reflex is a proprioceptive reflex obtained from the muscles of the neck and probably from the sense receptors of the ligaments and joints of the cervical spine. The reflex produces maximal extensor tone in the arm and leg of the side to which the face is turned (face limbs) and maximal flexor tone in the arm and leg of the opposite side (skull limbs). To elicit: place the individual in a supine position and turn his head to one side. The reflex is present at birth and is inhibited between approximately four months and one year.

Symmetrical Tonic Neck Reflex

The symmetrical tonic neck reflex is a proprioceptive reflex similarly obtained from the sense receptors of the neck, which produces extension of the arms and flexion of the legs when the head is raised and flexion of the arms and extension of the legs when the head is lowered. To elicit: place the individual over the knees, or in a crawling position if possible, raise or lower the head and test the arms and legs for flexor and extensor tone as indicated. The reflex appears at about two months and is inhibited between approximately four and twelve months.

Tonic Labyrinthine Reflex

The tonic labyrinthine reflex is evoked by changes in the position of the head in space, probably by stimulation of the otolith organs of the labyrinths. It produces maximal extensor tone in the supine position and maximal flexor tone in the prone position. To elicit: place the individual in the supine position and test the arms and legs for extensor tone; or, place the individual in the prone position and test the arms and legs for flexor tone. The reflex operates closely with the tonic neck reflex, appears sometime during the first two months of life and is inhibited between approximately four and twelve months.

Positive and Negative Supporting Reactions

The positive supporting reaction is characterized by the simultaneous contraction of flexors and extensors which exert a synergic action resulting in the fixation of the joints of the legs. This action is stimulated by contact of the pads of the feet with the ground which causes the stretching of the intrinsic muscles of the feet. To elicit: bounce the individual several times on the balls of his feet.

The negative supporting reaction is characterized by a reflex relaxation of the extensors of the proximal joints. To elicit: lift the individual off the ground after testing for the positive supporting reaction and evaluate the flexor tone of the limbs.

Associated Reactions

Associated reactions (Walshe, 1923, 1946) are released postural reactions which may produce a widespread increase of spasticity in all parts of the body. To elicit: have a hemiplegic squeeze an object with his sound hand; an increase in spasticity on the hemiplegic side is indicative of a positive response. With a quadriplegic patient there may be an increase in spasticity throughout the body when he attempts to move one limb.

It should be instructive to point out here that CNS evolution marked by brain stem sensorimotor integration only would not ordinarily allow the child to assume a quadrupedal crawling position.

Figure 2 shows how selected brain stem reflexes are elicited as well as the associated characteristic postures.

MIDBRAIN REFLEXES

Continuing the human, neuro-ontogenetic ascent we come to the midbrain reflexes. These reflexes are integrated at the level of the midbrain above the red nucleus. They interact with each other and work toward establishing a normal head and body relationship in space, as well as in relation to each other. Their combined action enables the child to roll over, to sit up, to get up on hands and knees, and to stand up. The righting reflexes develop in a definite sequence from birth onward and their appearance coincides with the recognized milestones of the child's motor development. As cortical control increases,

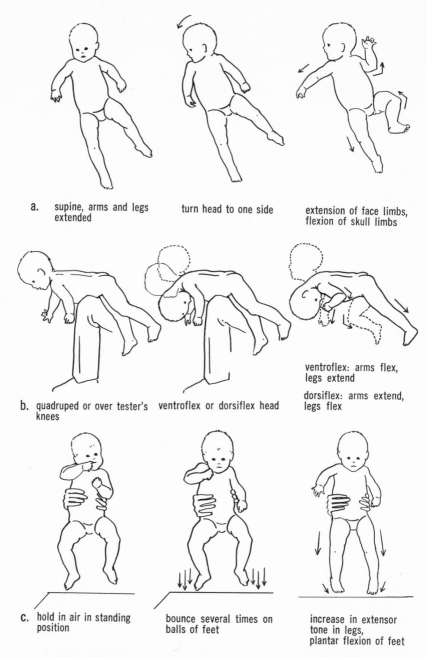

a. supine, arms and legs extended   turn head to one side   extension of face limbs, flexion of skull limbs

ventroflex: arms flex, legs extend

dorsiflex: arms extend, legs flex

b. quadruped or over tester's knees   ventroflex or dorsiflex head

c. hold in air in standing position   bounce several times on balls of feet   increase in extensor tone in legs, plantar flexion of feet

Figure 2. Brain stem reflexes: elicitation and characteristic posture.
a. asymmetrical tonic neck reflex. b. symmetrical tonic neck reflex.
c. positive supporting reaction.

16

they are gradually inhibited and disappear around the age of three to five years. They were studied by Magnus (1924, 1926).

Neck Righting Reflex

The neck righting reflex is evoked basically by stimulation of the neck proprioceptors. To elicit: turn the individual's head to one side; this should cause the rotation of the body as a whole toward the side to which the head is turned. The reflex is present at birth, is strong until four months, and diminishes thereafter. A lack of neck righting after one month or a persistent reaction after six months may be indicators of CNS dysmaturation.

Labyrinthine Righting Reflex Acting On The Head

The labyrinthine righting reflex acting on the head gradually emerges from the fourth to the sixth week onward. At first, the reaction is weak and the baby raises his head in the prone position between one and three months. Later, as he gains strength, the baby begins to raise his head in the supine position during the fourth to the sixth month. To elicit: blindfold the individual, hold him with both hands around the pelvis, and slowly move him through various positions in space, for example, upright, prone, supine, and sideways to the left and to the right. The individual should bring his head into the normal position, which is face vertical and mouth horizontal. The reaction in the prone position is present at about one to two months and in the supine at about six months; both continue throughout life. A lack of reaction in the prone after the second month and in the supine after the sixth month may indicate CNS dysmaturation.

Body Righting Reflex Acting On The Body

The body righting reflex acting on the body appears around the sixth to the eighth month and is not present after three years. It modifies the neck righting reaction by the addition of a rotation of the trunk between the shoulders and pelvis, that is, the head turns to one side, then the shoulder girdle, and finally the pelvis. The receptors include the tactile sense organs of the body surface. The body-righting-on-body reflex sequence is as follows: from ten to twelve months of age, the child uses a complete rotation pattern by turning over to his abdomen and getting on his hands and knees before sitting; between two and three and up to five years of age, the child uses a partial rotation pattern by leaning on one arm and then pushing up into the sitting position; and finally, after five years, the child sits up by using a symmetrical pattern.

Body Righting Reflex Acting On The Head

The body righting reflex acting on the head serves to right the head in response to some part of the body touching a supporting surface, for example, head righting will follow when the individual's feet touch the ground or when one side of the body is pressed against a hard surface. This reaction interacts closely with the labyrinthine righting reflex acting on the head to secure the normal position of the head in space. It appears at about four to six months and is inhibited between one to five years.

Optical Righting Reflex Acting On The Head

The optical righting reflex acting on the head is of secondary importance at first but gains quickly in influence as the child grows. The head follows movements of the eyes and hence the eyes contribute to head orientation. Testing is similar to the labyrinthine righting reflex acting on the head but with no blindfold. The reflex appears at around four weeks and remains active throughout life. In prone, the reaction appears at about one to two months; in supine at about six months; and in tilting from right to left from the upright at about six to eight months.

Amphibian Reaction

The amphibian reaction is a prerequisite to crawling. To elicit: place the individual in the prone position, and with the fingers apply pressure or lift in the pelvic area on one side. A positive response is marked by an automatic flexion of arm, hip, and knee on that side. The reaction may be observed at about six months and continues throughout life.

Figure 3 shows how selected midbrain reflexes are elicited as well as the sequence of movements involved.

EQUILIBRIUM REACTIONS

Completing the neuro-ontogenetic ascent toward sensorimotor integration centers which are responsible for progressively less organized, more complex, less automatic behavior, we arrive at the level of the equilibrium reactions.

These reactions are mediated by the efficient interaction of the cortex, basal ganglia, and cerebellum. The body proprioceptors are the main receptors; the labyrinths are active to a lesser degree. They occur only when muscle tone is normal or near normal, and they provide for body adaptation in response to a change in the center of gravity of the body. They may be seen to emerge from the age of about six months on, persist throughout life, and find their full development in the human organism. Also, it is known that a positive reaction at one motor level indicates that the next higher level of motor activity is possible. The full development of the equilibrium reactions brings the individual to the bipedal stage of motor development and, therefore, completes the description of human neuroevolution. These reactions were studied by various investigators, for example, Rademaker, 1935; Weisz, 1938; and Zador, 1938.

Supine and Prone Equilibrium Reaction

To elicit equilibrium reactions in supine or prone positions: place the individual on a tilt board and tilt him to one side. A positive reaction is marked by the bending of the head and the arching of the body toward the raised side and the abduction and extension of the arms and legs in protective and balance movements. In prone the reaction may first be noticed at about four to six months, and in supine about seven to ten months.

Side-Lying Equilibrium Reaction

To elicit equilibrium reactions in the side-lying position: place the individual on his side, abduct the free arm and raise him. A positive reaction is characterized by an angulation of the head toward the body on the raised side and abduction of the leg on the same side; in addition, there is abduction and extension of the arm on the opposite side as the individual is pulled to a sitting position.

Crawling Equilibrium Reaction

To elicit equilibrium reactions in the crawling position: place the individual in prone resting on his elbows ("puppy position") and tip the body to one side by raising one shoulder. Abduction and extension of the raised arm and leg to equalize the weight transference, and abduction of the opposite arm and leg as a protective reaction constitute a positive reaction. This "puppy position" represents the start of "two-point crawling" activity where the child uses both arms together to pull himself forward (one point), while he pushes with both legs together (second point).

Heel-Sitting Equilibrium Reaction

To elicit equilibrium reactions in the heel-sitting position: place the individual in the proper position and push gently to one side. A positive reaction is revealed by the arm and leg of the pushed side abducting and extending as a balance reaction, while the opposite arm abducts and extends as a protective reaction. This position represents the

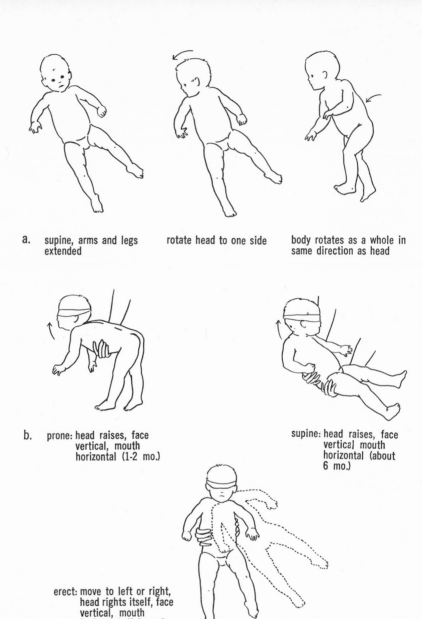

a.   supine, arms and legs   rotate head to one side   body rotates as a whole in
         extended   same direction as head

b.   prone: head raises, face   supine: head raises, face
              vertical, mouth   vertical mouth
              horizontal (1-2 mo.)   horizontal (about
                                                     6 mo.)

erect: move to left or right,
        head rights itself, face
        vertical, mouth
        horizontal (6-8 mo.)

Figure 3. Midbrain reflexes: elicitation and characteristic movement.
a. neck righting reflex. b. labyrinthine righting reflexes acting on head.

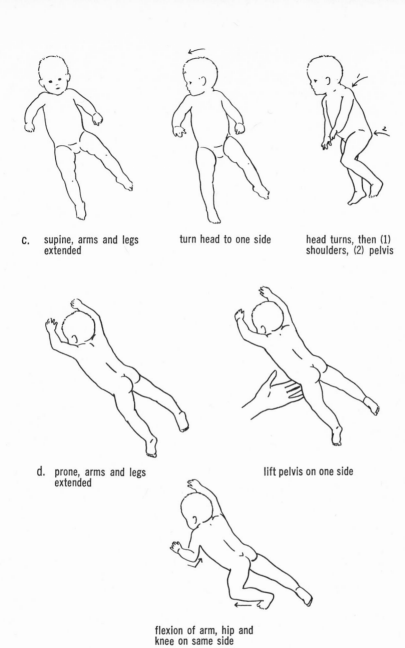

c. supine, arms and legs   turn head to one side   head turns, then (1)
    extended   shoulders, (2) pelvis

d. prone, arms and legs   lift pelvis on one side
    extended

flexion of arm, hip and
knee on same side

Figure 3. Midbrain reflexes: elicitation and characteristic movement.
c. body righting reflex acting on body. d. amphibian reaction.

start of "three-point crawling" activity where the child progresses by reciprocal movements of the arms (two points) in conjunction with a movement of both legs together (third point).

Quadrupedal Equilibrium Reaction

To elicit equilibrium reactions in the quadrupedal position: place the individual on all fours and tip gently to one side. A positive reaction is shown by the abduction and extension of the arm and leg on the raised side as a balance reaction, and the abduction of the opposite arm as a protective reaction; it appears at about ten to twelve months. This position represents the start of "four-point crawling" activity where the child progresses by reciprocating movements of both hands and both knees (four points).

Sitting Equilibrium Reaction

To elicit equilibrium reactions in the sitting position: place the individual on a chair or sitting surface, or a side-to-side rocking chair, and push gently to one side. A positive reaction is indicated when the head moves toward the raised side, the arm and leg of the raised side abduct and extend as a balance reaction; and the opposite arm and leg abduct and extend as a protective reaction; or push the individual backward and observe the head, shoulders, and arms move forward and the legs extend; or push the individual forward and observe the legs flex, the spine and neck extend, and the arms move backward. These reactions appear at about twelve to fourteen months.

Kneel-Standing Equilibrium Reaction

To elicit equilibrium reactions in the kneel-standing position: place the individual on his knees and pull to one side by holding an abducted and extended arm. A positive reaction is manifested by the abduction and extension of the opposite arm and leg, and the angulation of the head toward the body on the same side; or push the individual backward and observe the head, shoulders, and arms move forward as a balance reaction. The reaction appears at about thirteen to fifteen months. The kneel-standing position represents the starting position for kneel-walking activity where the child progresses by reciprocating movements of the knees.

* Simian Stance Equilibrium Reaction

To elicit equilibrium reactions in the simian stance position: place the individual in a crouched position with palm surfaces touching the floor between abducted knees and gently push to one side. A positive

---

* This posture was first described and utilized by the author during the pilot studies described in Chapter Three.

reaction is indicated by the abduction and extension of the raised side as a balance reaction, and the abduction and extension of the opposite arm as a protective reaction. Children who are learning to stand may be seen to use this posture and progress in it for a short space before rising. The reaction may be observed at about fifteen to eighteen months and continues throughout life.

Head, Trunk, and Arm Equilibrium Reaction

To elicit equilibrium reactions of the head, trunk, and arms: place the individual in a standing position, hold by the pelvis, knees, or ankles (depending on amount of support required by the individual to maintain the standing position), and rotate, tip from side-to-side, or move forward and backward. A positive reaction is reflected by balance reactions of the head, trunk, and arms in order to maintain equilibrium.

Standing Equilibrium Reaction

To elicit equilibrium reactions in standing: place the individual in an erect position and pull to one side by holding an abducted and extended arm. A positive reaction is marked by the abduction and extension of the opposite arm and leg as a balance reaction and the righting of the head to maintain the normal position in space. Or hold the individual under the axillae and tip him backward; this causes the head, shoulders, and arms to move forward and the feet to dorsiflex. These reactions appear at about twelve to eighteen months.

See-Saw Equilibrium Reaction

To elicit see-saw equilibrium reactions: place the individual in a standing position, hold the arm in extension and the leg of the same side in flexion (foot in palm of tester's hand), and gently pull the person toward you. A positive response is marked by a strong extension and abduction of that leg, plus righting and balance reactions of the head, arms, and thorax. The reaction may be observed at about fifteen months and continues throughout life.

Hopping Equilibrium Reaction

To elicit hopping equilibrium reactions: place the individual in a standing position, hold him under the axillae and move him from side to side, forward, and backward. A positive reaction is shown when the person attempts to keep his balance and support his body by making sideways, or forward, or backward steps in the direction of the weight transference. Such reactions may be observed at about fifteen to eighteen months.

Figure 4 shows how various equilibrium reactions are elicited and the characteristic sequence of movements involved.

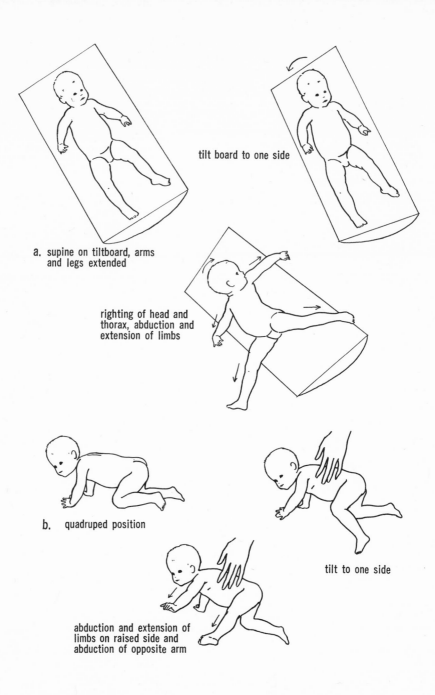

tilt board to one side

a. supine on tiltboard, arms and legs extended

righting of head and thorax, abduction and extension of limbs

b. quadruped position

tilt to one side

abduction and extension of limbs on raised side and abduction of opposite arm

Figure 4. Equilibrium reactions: elicitation and characteristic movements. a. supine equilibrium reaction. b. quadrupedal equilibrium reaction.

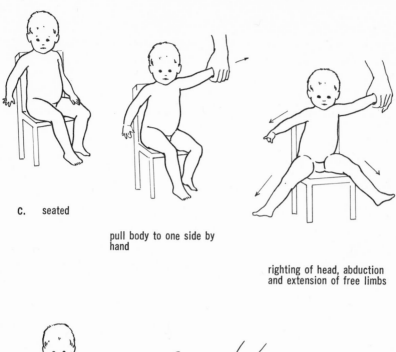

c. seated

pull body to one side by hand

righting of head, abduction and extension of free limbs

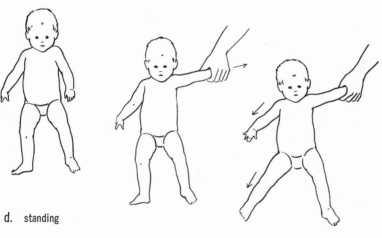

d. standing

pull body to one side by hand

righting of head, abduction and extension of opposite limbs

Figure 4. Equilibrium reactions: elicitation and characteristic movements. c. sitting equilibrium reaction. d. standing equilibrium reaction.

ADDITIONAL MOVEMENT REFLEXES AND REACTIONS

In addition to the more easily categorized reflexes and reactions described here are a group that may be called the movement responses. Many of these responses will be referred to in the chapter on neurotherapy procedures.

Moro Reflex

The Moro reflex (Magnus, 1926) is strong during the first three months of life, becomes weaker, and finally disappears at about six months of age. It can be elicited by a number of stimuli such as sudden noise, movement of the supporting surface, tapping of the abdomen, blowing on the face, and tipping the individual backward. A positive reaction is an abductor-extensor reaction of various parts of the body; following this, the arms may be seen to return to the more usual flexed position.

Startle Reflex

The startle reflex (McGraw, 1962, p. 19) represents a reversal of the Moro reflex with the positive response being one of an adductor-flexor reaction of various body parts; it may be seen in older children and adults who are startled or surprised.

Landau Reflex

The Landau reflex (Schaltenbrand, 1927; Byers, 1938) is a combination of tonic and righting reflexes. It appears at about the age of six months and disappears by two or three years of age. To elicit: hold the individual prone in the air and support by one hand under the thorax. A positive response is noted when the individual first lifts the head so that the face is in the vertical position (due to the righting reflexes on the head); this is then followed by a tonic extension of the spine and legs (due to the influence of the symmetrical tonic neck reflex).

Protective-Extensor-Thrust of the Arms (PET)

The PET of the arms reflex (Schaltenbrand, 1927) starts at about four months, is strong at six months of age, and remains active throughout adult life. To elicit: place the individual in a prone position, lift him freely in the air by his ankles and move suddenly downward. Or with an older person, place him in a prone position, raise his body off the floor by holding onto the pelvis and then move him downward. A positive response is marked by an immediate extension of the arms with abduction and extension of the fingers.

Upper Limb Movement

In discussing the examination of the newborn, Thomas described an infantile upper limb movement (1960, p. 21) which should be of interest here. To elicit: place the infant or child in the prone and extend upper limbs alongside the trunk. A positive response consists of head turning, flexion of arms and forearms and a moving forward of the upper limbs (facilitated by tactile stimulation of the hands). Towards the end of the first month the baby can raise his head slightly and by about three months he can hold the erect head position well; also at about three months he can support himself on his forearms, thus raising his thorax and head.

Primary Walking

Automatic or primary walking activity in the newborn was also described by Thomas (1960, p. 31). To elicit: hold the newborn upright with feet on the ground and gently move him in a forward direction. A positive response includes walking movements with good coordination and regular rhythm, but without balancing or associated movements of the upper limbs. The reaction does not occur backwards. It may be observed up to several weeks.

Precipitation Reflex

The precipitation reflex was described by Rademaker and may be observed at about six to eight months. To elicit: hold the baby by his trunk and move downwards and sideways. A positive response consists of upper limb extension (including fingers) towards the table in a seeking-for-support pattern. The pattern appears before actual contact is made by the upper limbs. The limb supporting activity is strong enough to support the body weight; each limb can be evaluated separately.

Placing Response of Upper Limb

The placing reaction of the upper limb has been described by Thomas (1960, p. 39). To elicit: hold the infant upright and apply back of one hand to the under edge of a table. The first stage of a positive reaction consists of upper limb flexion which brings the hand above the table. The second stage which consists of limb extension in a supporting movement (the supporting action of the upper limb takes place first with the use of the fist, and later on with the use of an open palm) occurs at about the third or fourth month.

Primary Sitting

Infantile passive and spontaneous sitting reactions have been described by Thomas (1960, p. 41). To elicit: pull the infant by his hands from supine to sitting. During the first few weeks the posture is accomplished with a head lag. At about three months, the head assumes a more normal position; however, the baby still takes no active part in the total movement. Near the end of the first six months, only a slight pull by the hands is needed to elicit the primary sitting pattern.

Placing Response of Lower Limb

To elicit the placing response of the lower limb (Prechtl and Beintema, 1964, p. 53), the infant is raised and the dorsum of one foot is lightly touched against the edge of the table. The first stage of a positive reaction consists of lower limb flexion which brings the lower limb above the table; the second stage consists of limb extension upon contact of the sole of the foot with the table. The reaction may be observed after the first ten days of life.

Definitive Walking

Definitive infantile walking has been described by Thomas (1960, p. 45). Slowly, after several weeks, primary walking activity changes. There is increasing use of toe-tips, and speed, rhythm, and coordination diminish. During the period of transition from primary to definitive walking, that is, between about the second and sixth months, the feet begin to drag and near the end of the period the infant tends to jump or to beat the floor with the feet in an alternating fashion.

At about the sixth or seventh month, the stage of definitive walking emerges and the infant again takes steps if he is lifted and pushed along. These first steps do not show the coordination characteristic of primary walking. The sequence of foot contact with the ground is first by the toes, then by the whole sole, and later the heel touches first.

Related to the phenomena associated with transition from primary to definitive walking are statements by McGraw (1962, p. 23) on neonatal neuromuscular behavior. McGraw indicated that the course of development in each function represents

> . . . a period during which the behavior reflects further maturation of subcortical or nuclear mechanisms; a period of diminution in overt expression, which seemingly reflects the onset of cortical inhibition upon the functioning of nuclear centers; the invasion of cortical control over the function, as indicated by the deliberate or voluntary quality of overt activity; and, finally, the integration of the various neural centers involved in a function, as evidenced by a smooth, frictionless type of performance.

Arm Walking

During the second to sixth month period and before the appearance of spontaneous crawling, a tendency toward rhythmic progression of the arms might be observed. To elicit: hold child up by the trunk and legs and move the child in a forward direction. The initial response is usually a forward movement on forearms with clenched fists; eventually the arms and fingers extend and alternating movements of the arms gradually improve.

Spontaneous and Reinforced Crawling

Spontaneous crawling and crawling with reinforcement may be observed in the newborn infant (Prechtl and Beintema, 1964, p. 48). To elicit: place the infant in the prone and wait for about half a minute. A positive response (likely after the first three or four days of life) is spontaneous crawling movements. A reinforcing stimulus, that is, pressing hands gently on the soles of the feet may increase crawling movements and may actually cause some movement of the baby (Bauer's Response).

Bowing Reflex

Peiper (1963, p. 171) has described the bowing reflex which was originally reported by Gamper. To elicit: apply pressure to lower limbs or extend thighs at the hip joints with child in the supine. The positive response consists of head and neck ventroflexion, followed by ventroflexion of the trunk; the child eventually assumes a sitting position with a curved back. The sitting position is accomplished by frequent sideward turns of the head and trunk. The reflex can occasionally be elicited in healthy premature infants.

Chain Reflexes

Symmetrical and asymmetrical chain reflexes, which are dependent on the labyrinthine righting reflex acting on the head, have been studied by Peiper (1963, pp. 180–191). "As soon as the infant succeeds in righting his head in space, his whole body tries by means of reflexes to adjust to this position. Chain reflexes starting from the head regulate the position of the neck, trunk, arms, pelvis, and legs down to the tips of the toes in order to maintain equilibrium."

Chain reflexes, or synreflexic responses, can be elicited in various positions and it is believed that neck and body righting reflexes and tonic neck and labyrinthine righting reflexes contribute to the formation of the various types of chain reflexes. Two will be described here.

Symmetrical Chain Reflex in the Abdominal Position. To elicit the symmetrical chain reflex in the abdominal position: place the child in prone on a table, move his head and thorax forward over the edge of the table so that only the pelvis remains supported by the table (tester holds child in the area of the upper thighs). A positive response consists of upward arching of the head and trunk, and simultaneous raising and sideways stretching and flexing at the elbows of both arms. The reflex gradually appears during the first month of life and disappears at about two years.

Asymmetrical Chain Reflex in the Suspended Oblique Lateral Position. To elicit the asymmetrical chain reflex in the suspended oblique lateral position: raise the child in a suspended oblique lateral position with his head up and supported in the region of the waist. A positive response consists of head righting, followed by righting of the upper half of the body, arching of the body, and extension of the upper limbs and some flexing of the lower limbs. If the body is moved from the right oblique to the left oblique, the head remains righted while the extremities change their positions. The reflex appears during the fourth to sixth months of life.

Figure 5 shows how some of these reflexes and reactions are elicited and the sequence of movements involved.

After a careful study of human neurodevelopment, it is hoped the reader will find the material in the succeeding chapters, which is basically devoted to explaining principles and methods of neurotherapy, easier to understand and to integrate.

REFERENCES

Byers, R. K. "Tonic neck reflexes in children," *Am. J. Dis. Child.,* 55 (1938), 696–742.

Magnus, R. "Some results of studies in the physiology of posture," *Lancet,* 2 (1926), 531–535.

Magnus, R. *Koerperstellung.* Berlin: Springer, 1924.

McGraw, Myrtle, B. *The Neuromuscular Maturation of the Human Infant.* New York: Hafner Publishing Co., 1962.

Prechtl, H. and Beintema, D. *The Neurological Examination of the Full Term Newborn Infant.* London: William Heinemann Medical Books Ltd., 1964.

Rademaker, G. *Reactions Labyrinthiques et Equilibre.* Paris: Masson et Cie, 1935.

Schaltenbrand, G. "The development of human motility and motor disturbances," *Arch. Neur. and Psych.,* 20 (1928), 720–730.

Sherrington, C. S. *Selected Writings* in D. Denny-Brown (Ed.). London: Hamish Hamilton Medical Books, 1939.

Sherrington, C. S. *The Integrative Action of the Nervous System*. London: Cambridge University Press, 1947.

Thomas, A. *et al. The Neurological Examination of the Infant*. London: National Spastics Soc., 1960.

Walshe, F. M. R. "On certain tonic or postural reflexes in hemiplegia with special reference to the so-called associated movements," *Brain*, 46 (1923), 1–37.

Walshe, F. M. R. *On the Contribution of Clinical Study to the Physiology of the Cerebral Cortex*. The Victor Horsley Memorial Lecture. Edinburgh: G. & S. Livingstone, Ltd., 1946.

Weisz, S. "Studies in equilibrium reaction," *J. Nerv. Ment. Dis.*, 88 (1938), 150–162.

Zador, J. *Les Reactions d'Equilibre Chez l'Homme*. Paris: Masson et Cie, 1938.

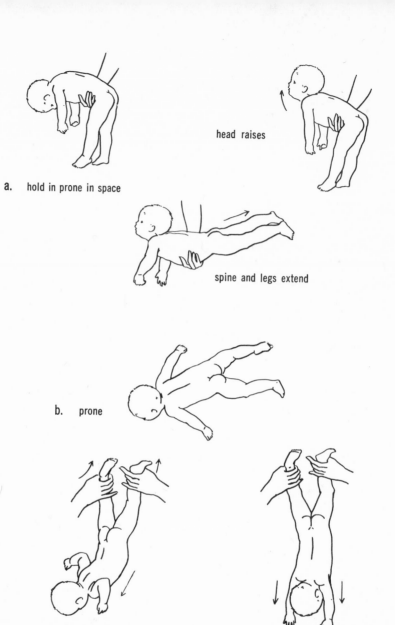

a. hold in prone in space

head raises

spine and legs extend

b. prone

lift freely in air by ankles
and move suddenly
downwards

arms extend, fingers extend
and abduct

Figure 5. Movement reflexes and reactions: elicitation and characteristic
movements.
a. Landau reflex. b. protective-extensor-thrust of the arms reaction.

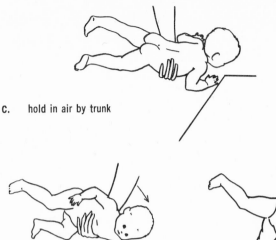

c.   hold in air by trunk

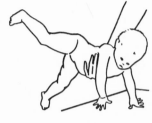

move downwards and
sideways

limb extends and supports
body weight

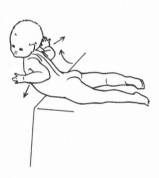

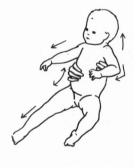

d.   abdominal position

suspended oblique lateral
position

Figure 5. Movement reflexes and reactions: elicitation and characteristic
   movements.
   c. precipitation reflex. d. symmetrical and asymmetrical chain reflexes.

33

Neurotherapy Procedures

Chapter Three will be concerned with the following: (1) presenting therapy methods and techniques based on neuroevolutional concepts; (2) offering a rationale for the methods and techniques cited; (3) outlining needs in establishing neurotherapy programs; and (4) presenting the results of a study of the application of neurotherapy procedures.

RATIONALE

Prior to beginning the discussion of the rationale for neurotherapy, some mention should be made of the role played by types of cerebral palsy in planning neurotherapy programs. In this regard, recent comments by Twitchell (1965) reflect rather well the view held by the author.

Twitchell states that ". . . from the neurophysiological view, the separation of patients into various categories—such as spasticity, rigidity, athetosis, tremor—is wholly artificial." He goes on to say that regardless of classification, the physiological substrata for spasticity and for athetotic phenomena, as examples, can be demonstrated in all patients. "Strict adherence to the various classifications of cerebral palsy are artificial and based on unphysiological tenets."

Twitchell also indicated that the defect in voluntary movement and in reflex mechanisms in cerebral palsy have a common basis which ". . . is a defect in sensory-motor integration with conflict between hypertrophied infantile reflexes." He urges that ". . . more attention be paid to the physiological basis for the motor deficit in each individual patient so that treatment could be oriented to that individual patient rather than to some arbitrary grouping."

Returning to the discussion of rationale, it is proposed that neurotherapy is fundamentally a tactile-proprioceptive approach designed to suppress spinal, and brain stem nervous centers and activate midbrain (righting reactions) and midbrain plus cortical and cerebellar centers (equilibrium reactions). Using Jacksonian terminology, the goal in therapy is to stimulate the process of nervous evolution starting from the particular child's level of nervous system arrestment, retardation, or dissolution. That is, one attempts to change the child's motor patterns from most reflex, or most organized and most automatic (infantile), to least reflex, or least organized and least automatic (mature), by employing techniques which will (1) progressively inhibit lower centers of sensorimotor integration and thereby fractionate the infantile postures and movements and normalize muscle tone (reducing positive symptoms); and (2) progressively shunt sensory inflow to higher centers of sensorimotor integration and thereby elicit more mature postures, movements, and muscle tone (reducing negative symptoms). In line with this goal is Jackson's statement (1958, p. 91), "What on the lowest level are centres for simplest movements of the limbs become evolved in the highest centres into the physical bases of volition."

The "stimulation-development" principle of emergent reflexes and reactions is a general principle which may explain best why neurophysiologic therapy techniques may be effective. This principle applies to the stimulation of desired reflexes and reactions which have not developed, or have been lost, as well as to the weakening of abnormally retained or released infantile reflexes and reactions. According to this principle, motor responses which emerge as a function of maturation may be facilitated by proper provocation, unless the type and extent of nervous system damage precludes it. On the other hand, extinction of undesired motor responses, which are supposed to disappear as a function of maturation, is accomplished basically by applying the adequate stimulus and then aborting the expected response (Mysak, 1963). That certain primitive responses can be suppressed in affected children in this manner has been demonstrated in a film of a pilot study (Mysak, 1960).

NEUROPHYSIOLOGICAL CONSIDERATIONS IN DEVELOPING THERAPY PROCEDURES

In addition to neuroevolutional concepts, certain other neurophysiological data have been utilized to good advantage in developing neurotherapy procedures and in giving these procedures support. A discussion of these ideas follows.

Reflexive Maturation Determines Motor Development

The development of various motor activities—such as head-raising, side-lying, sitting, standing, walking—depends on the combination of reflexive mechanism maturation and afferent stimulation (e.g., that stimulation received during rocking, and handling during feeding, changing, dressing, bathing, and play periods). This combination excites a great deal of automatic movement in the form of righting and equilibrium reactions; and these movement patterns contribute to the development of these emerging motor activities. Therefore, it would appear logical that shifting the focus of therapy from directly teaching volitional and refined motor activities to attempting to stimulate neuromaturation and automatic movement reactions should prove of value in cerebral palsy habilitation.

The table in Appendix A illustrates the relationship between reflexive maturation and the development of certain motor activities in the normal child. For example, head raising in the prone position, which takes place at from one to three months, waits upon the emergence of the labyrinthine righting reflex acting on the head, which is manifested at about two months; sitting, which takes place at about eight to ten months, waits upon the emergence of the body righting reflex acting on the body, which is manifested between seven and twelve months. Similar relationships between background reflexes and reactions and oral and hand activities are also shown in Appendix A.

In short, the clinical lesson to be learned here is that prior to teaching volitional and refined motor activities to cerebral palsied children, the clinician should first attempt to stimulate the necessary background reflexive maturation and to elicit appropriate automatic movement patterns.

Stimulating Higher-Order Sensorimotor Integration

Another neurophysiologic concept which contributes to the development of therapy procedures is the concept of levels of sensorimotor integration. Following are some ideas connected with the problem of lower-center sensorimotor integration and with ways of shunting sensory inflow to higher centers.

Afferent "Short-Circuiting." Because of pathologically-released domination over sensorimotor systems by spinal and brain stem levels (due to arrestment, retardation, or dissolution of the CNS), the abnormal motor patterns of many cerebral-palsied children may be seen as the result of "short-circuiting" of afferent inflow into lower-order synaptic channels (positive symptoms or reflections of infantile sensorimotor integration). It is believed that such a condition prevents the child from utilizing higher, possibly intact sensorimotor integration centers. To state this in another way, released infantile brain centers may be "draining off" sensory inflow, thus preventing the inflow from reaching higher centers and not allowing the child to manifest all of his sensorimotor potential. Therefore, if such a situation exists in the cerebral palsied, therapy techniques designed to encourage afferent integration at higher centers should prove useful.

Afferent Inflow Determines Efferent Outflow. The utilization of Magnus' (1924) "law of shunting" offers a way of counteracting the sensory "short-circuiting" just described. It has been hypothesized that the state of contraction and elongation of muscles determines the distribution of excitatory and inhibitory processes within the CNS and, therefore, the subsequent efferential outflow (afferent inflow favors the contraction of elongated muscles). The implication here is that the clinician by manipulating the body musculature in various ways, may differentially influence the distribution of excitatory and inhibitory processes within the CNS. In other words, the clinician may be able to activate or "open" higher sensory pathways within the child's CNS and hence effect new motor outflows.

Unmanifested Efferent Potential. In addition, because of sensory "short-circuiting" and the frequently associated increased muscle tone, potentially-present and higher-integrated righting and equilibrium reactions may not be seen (these reactions emerge adequately only when muscle tone is normal or at least near normal). That is, centers for higher-order motor patterns which may not be damaged are nevertheless prevented from manifesting themselves not only because of sensory "short-circuiting" but also because of heightened muscle tone. This suggests that if ways could be devised to at least improve the state of the child's general muscle tone, some of this unmanifested efferent potential might emerge.

Stimulation and "Rutting" of Sensorimotor Patterns. Finally, it has been stated by Russell (1958) that there is a tendency for nerve cells to repeat patterns of activity, and that this tendency is apparently one of the most powerful features of all nervous functioning. In addition, as higher nervous arrangements are activated in the CNS, they not only provide for more differentiated motor patterns but they also exert inhibitory controls over lower, previously dominant motor centers. These statements suggest that if new and higher-order automatic movement patterns can be stimulated by certain neurotherapy techniques, especially if these are normally-emerging motor patterns such as righting and equilibrium reactions, they may be "rutted in" (physiological memory) and made part of an individual's motor repertoire by virtue of repetition of evocation.

Reducing Secondary Sensorimotor Deficits

The sensorium, as has already been brought out, is crucial to motor activities; for example, sensory deficits may affect (1) motor development, because motor acts are not learned but only their associated sensations; (2) motor monitoring, because proprioceptors are essential in the guidance of movements excited by the exteroceptors; and (3) body-image development, because adequate development depends to a certain degree on the integration of sensory inflow resulting from moving normally. The latter development is important to future sensory-perceptual-symbolic maturation. Depending on the degree of primary sensory loss in any given neuropathology, all the above factors may be disturbed to various degrees. However, in cerebral palsy, these factors may be disturbed further because of secondary sensory involvements.

Secondary sensory aberrations may result either from the "short-circuiting" of inflow, from the distortion of inflow because sensory receptors may be in abnormally-toned muscle environments, or from anxiety-induced delays in sensory feedback. This suggests that procedures which tend to regularize muscle tone and encourage higher-center integration of sensory inflow could reduce the effects of the secondary sensory deficits, and, therefore, tend to reduce the apparent severity of the over-all cerebral palsy problem.

The above discussion should indicate that the utilization of certain neurophysiological data may not only contribute to a better understanding of cerebral palsy and its symptoms, but also contribute to the development of fruitful neurophysiologically-based therapy concepts.

To summarize the therapy implications of this section of the chapter, it has been suggested that the child with cerebral palsy might be helped if his body musculature could be manipulated in a manner that would regularize his muscle tone and positively influence the distribution of excitatory and inhibitory processes within his CNS; if, consequently, he could actualize his usually greater potential for higher kinds of automatic motor movements; and, finally, of course, if these newly-emerged automatic movements could be maintained by repetition (physiology of memory) and eventually utilized in the development of various desired volitional and more complex motor activities.

The following sections of the chapter deal with types of neurotherapy programs, program considerations, and a review of a study of the application of neurophysiological therapy techniques.

NEUROTHERAPY PROGRAMS

Depending on the severity of the child's neurological disorder and on the amount of positive symptomatology, developmental neurotherapy may take at least three forms. It should be understood that only the basic principles and procedures of these three forms will be presented here. More specific techniques should be developed by the clinician after a careful study of the individual child's neurophysiological disorder.

Type I: Facilitation of Normal Development of Reflexes and Reactions

The Type I or Facilitatory Approach is designed for young or mildly involved children and the emphasis is placed on exciting normal automatic movements, and on providing environmental enrichment in the development of sensorimotor responses.

Planned excitation of the sensorium designed to facilitate head-raising, side-lying, sitting, standing, and so on, in about the normal sequence and at about the expected times, forms the nucleus of the approach. After assessing the child's level of nervous system evolution, the following reflexes and reactions should be stimulated at least twice a day: neck righting, labyrinthine righting reflex acting on the head, the body righting reflexes, amphibian reaction, protective-extensor-thrust of the arms reaction, primary sitting and walking, the precipitation reflex, arm-walking, reinforced crawling, and the chain reflexes. In addition, equilibrium reactions in all appropriate positions should also be elicited. Special attention should be paid to affected limbs so that they are guided to participate in the expected movements and postures as well as possible; techniques such as timed (with respect to time of expected response) placing, holding, extending, flexing, abducting, adducting, and so on, of the limbs should be planned.

Encouraging normal respiratory patterns is also recommended. (Respiratory techniques will be described in Chapter Five.)

These procedures when begun early should serve to keep muscle tone more normal, encourage the development of a more normal body image, and guide the child to engage in movements and assume postures in a more normal manner.

Also appropriate here are ideas expressed by Twitchell (1965) relative to the importance of environmental stimulation, or "environmental enrichment or deprivation" in the development of sensory-motor responses. For example, (1) the low threshold at birth for the instinctive sucking response remains at this low level only if the infant is immediately allowed to suck; (2) infants who sleep in the prone position usually develop sitting, standing, and walking more quickly than infants who sleep in supine, and this is apparently due to the more constant stimulation of righting reflexes resulting from body contact in the prone; (3) infants who are usually placed in standing postures on their mother's lap, thus restimulating the positive supporting reactions, usually begin to stand and walk earlier than those who are not; and, finally, (4) such "environmental enrichment" also appears to hasten spontaneous prehension in the developing infant.

Type I activities may be seen as both prophylactic and facilitatory, designed to stimulate and guide the affected child toward the highest possible level of nervous system evolution.

Type II: Positive Symptom Inhibition and Facilitation of Higher-Order Sensorimotor Reactions

The Type II or Inhibitory-Facilitatory Approach is for more involved children and employs three basic procedures. It has been discussed previously in an article describing the Bobath approach (Mysak, 1959). The goals were described as motor desynthesis, or the weakening of lower brain center domination over the CNS; motor elaboration, or the stimulation of higher brain center activity, and hence higher kinds of motor reactions; and motor resynthesis, or the use of these new and more complicated motor reactions in the development of more advanced volitional motor activity.

Level of Nervous System Evolution. The first step in the Type II approach involves the careful study of the child's movements, postures, and muscle tone in order to determine the child's level of nervous system evolution. The evaluation should indicate how dominant are the child's spinal and brain stem sensorimotor integration centers and the status of the child's righting and equilibrium reactions. For example, the analysis might reveal that the child is basically at a brain stem plus midbrain level of neurological development. (See Appendix B for a sample evaluation form.)

Positive Symptom Inhibition. On the basis of the above analysis, body postures contributive to positive symptom inhibition are planned. Concepts related to inhibiting postures are as follows: Inhibiting postures basically represent reversals of abnormal postures which tend to counteract retained or released spinal and brain stem reflexes as well as the frequently associated abnormal muscle tone; this special positioning with its concomitant muscle tone normalization appears to allow for a higher integration of sensory inflow. Four phases may be associated with these reversals of abnormal postures. The first phase is characterized by heightened tone in the muscles being elongated; the second phase is characterized by a reduction in muscle tone when the tendency for the elongated muscles to return to their former position is resisted by the clinician; the third phase is characterized by a gradual increase in tone following a certain period of normal or near-normal muscle tone; and the fourth phase is characterized by another return to more normal muscle tone when the third phase is again resisted.

Repetition of this procedure may be found to cause gradual lengthening of the periods of desired muscle tone. Depending on the treatment status of the child, these postures may first be imposed upon and gradually tolerated by the child (externally influenced inhibition), then eventually maintained (internally influenced inhibition), and, finally, assumed by the child (new volitional movements). It should be noted that these postures usually represent bodily attitudes from which new movements may be initiated, and may also represent intermediate steps from one motor position to the next higher one.

Facilitation of Higher-Order Sensorimotor Integration. Following the successful application of positive-symptom inhibiting postures, and during the periods of appropriate muscle tone, facilitation techniques are employed. The goal of these techniques is to obtain spontaneous movement responses from the child by special stimulation; for example, by exciting neck proprioceptors, or by exciting the otoliths by shifting the center of gravity of the body. The sensory inflow thus provided is apparently integrated at higher centers because, when successful, facilitation techniques often elicit higher types of reactions and hence new and desired movements and postures. In order to maintain these new postures, equilibrium reactions must be evoked at each higher level achieved. Assimilation of these higher-order movements, postures, and balance reactions, or the firm establishment of higher-order sensorimotor synaptic bonds, is accomplished basically by repetition of activity.

Examples of Application of Type II Approach. Let us suppose that the analysis of the child's level of neurological evolution reveals that he is basically a supine or prone-lying creature who is unable to raise his head in the prone position (negative symptoms) and that he also shows, for example, spinal reflexes, tonic labyrinthine reflexes, symmetrical and asymmetrical tonic neck reflexes, the positive supporting reaction, associated reactions, and the Moro reflex (positive symptoms).

With such findings, the clinician realizes that he is dealing with a child who is at an early infantile level of nervous system evolution. Therefore, one of the clinician's first goals might be to stimulate the labyrinthine righting reflex acting on the head in the prone position so that the child would be able to raise his head when lying on his stomach.

Close inspection may indicate that when the child is in the prone position, one of his positive symptoms, that is, the tonic labyrinthine reflex in the prone position, characterized by an increase in flexor tone throughout the body including the neck, is preventing the higher-integrated head righting reflex from emerging.

Attempts at stimulating CNS evolution from this early point begin by first weakening the tonic labyrinthine reflex. This is done by "disturbing" the sensorimotor circuitry associated with the tonic labyrinthine reflex in the prone; that is, the clinician should disturb the pattern which includes (1) sensory impulses from the labyrinths to the brain stem centers signaling the prone position of the child; (2) motor impulses emanating from brain stem centers and resulting in a general increase in flexor tone; and (3) sensory impulses feeding back and confirming the increase in flexor tone throughout the body and tending to strengthen the chain synaptic arrangement representing the tonic labyrinthine reflex acting in the prone position.

An attempt to disturb this sensorimotor pattern may be made by mismatching motor outflow and sensory feedback patterns; that is, the clinician modifies the flexor-adductor-inward rotation muscle pattern to an extensor-abductor-outward rotation muscle pattern and thereby feeds back to the CNS an incongruent sensory pattern.

Such a procedure is usually marked by resistance and a rise in muscle tone; however, if the clinician does not allow the muscles to return to their former posture, muscle tone may gradually lessen and something like near-normal muscle tonus may be appreciated—at least for a short time. By the effective use of this procedure, the clinician succeeds in imposing a sensory feedback pattern which is more appropriate to higher-center sensorimotor integration and he hopes that if these centers are reasonably intact they may begin to respond. Next, with the child in a posture which is preparatory for higher-center integration of sensory inflow, the clinician attempts to facilitate the emergence of the labyrinthine righting reflex acting on the head. This is done by holding the child's wrists and gently pulling until the shoulder girdle is raised, and then gently shaking the shoulder girdle and head in order to stimulate the labyrinths. If the positive symptom inhibiting posture has actually disturbed lower-center sensorimotor integration and is actually serving to provide sensory feedback appropriate to higher-center integration, the sensory inflow provided by stimulation of the otolith organs may, even at initial attempts at such procedures, evoke head-righting in the prone position. Establishment of these higher-order sensorimotor synaptic bonds is accomplished basically by repetition of activity. When the facilitation procedure in this instance has been successful, the clinician has in fact not only weakened the positive symptoms but has reduced the negative symptoms, in other words, he has stimulated the process of neuroevolution of human head position and functioning.

As a second example, it might be noted that a particular individual is unable to achieve side-lying from a supine position because of the effects of the tonic labyrinthine reflex acting in the supine position, which is marked by an increase in generalized extensor tone. In addition, when the child turns his head as an initial step in side-lying the asymmetrical tonic neck reflex may also be manifested. Both conditions make side-lying a difficult task. In this case, the positive symptom inhibiting posture may include: head ventroflexion, gentle flexing of the arms, and hip and knee flexion and abduction. Once inhibition has been established, side-lying is facilitated by lateralizing the head, thus stimulating neck proprioceptors and exciting the neck righting reflex.

It is hoped that these short examples of Type II treatment, with their accompanying explanations, have helped clarify the rationale underlying the neuroevolutional approach. They should also have made it clear to the reader that individuals who desire to learn to apply such techniques require training and experience before they may hope to become effective clinicians. Further clarification of the therapy rationale may be gained by presenting a diagram-description of the Type II approach.

Figure 6 shows at least three sources of possible afferent inflow that may excite movement: radiant energy via the eye (e.g., such energy may be responsible for the optical righting reflex acting on the head); sound pressure energy via the ear (e.g., such energy may be responsible for eliciting the Moro reflex or the startle reaction); and mechanical energy via the tactile and proprioceptive end organs (e.g., such energy may elicit the asymmetrical tonic neck reflexes and the body righting reflexes).

The diagram also shows levels along the neuraxis responsible for progressively higher sensorimotor integration (SMI). The four levels indicated coincide with integration centers at the spinal, brain stem, thalamic, and complete CNS levels, respectively. Further, the inhibitory (INH) functions of these centers are also illustrated. It is shown that as afferent inflow is integrated at successively higher centers along the neuraxis at least two phenomena occur. First, the center or centers immediately below the dominant integration center are inhibited and, second, a higher-order efferent outflow (M-1-4) is manifested. An additional example of neuroevolutional facilitation utilizing Figure 6 follows.

Let us suppose a seven-year-old cerebral palsied child is in a seated position and is subsequently tipped laterally in order to observe his reaction to having his body's center of gravity shifted. We may find that his reaction consists of an infantile flexor posture of the arms accompanied by finger extension and abduction and loss of sitting bal-

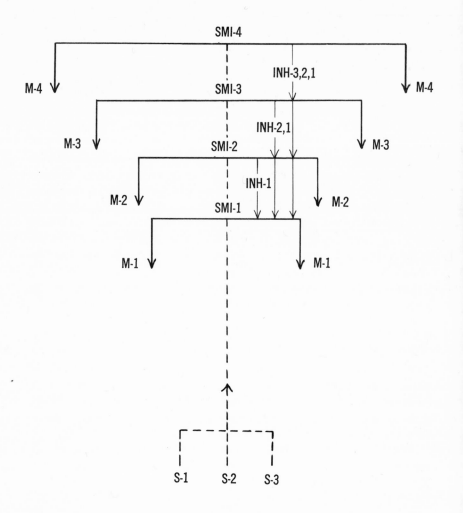

Figure 6. Schema of neurodynamics of progressively higher sensorimotor integration.

ance. In terms of the diagram, we may assume that the afferent inflow was integrated at the brain stem level (SMI-2) and hence infantile motor reactions were manifested (M-2).

The goal in therapy would be to interfere with the lower-order efferent outflow by preventing the infantile arm-hand reaction, thereby mismatching efferent outflow and afferent feedback patterns which, in turn, should disturb the functioning of the lower-order integration center. As the muscle tone which would have contributed to the infantile arm-hand posture subsides (inhibition), and tipping of the body is continued, the afferent inflow may now be shunted to higher centers (SMI-3,4) and equilibrium and righting reactions (M-3,4) in the sitting position may be manifested.

In summary, the following neurodynamics may be assumed during the successful application of the above procedures: afferent inflow reaches higher levels of sensorimotor integration (SMI-3,4) and the stimulation of these centers, in turn, inhibits the centers below it (INH-2,1) and provides efferent outflow which manifests itself in the form of higher-order righting and equilibrium reactions (M-3,4).

Type III: Positive Symptom Inhibition and Body Part Differentiation

When weakening of lower-order reflexes is progressing slowly, or not at all, and, consequently, is impeding the Type II approach to the problem, non-facilitatory techniques alone, or in combination with the Type II approach, may be employed. There are three aspects to the Inhibitory-Differentiation-Adaptation Approach.

Positive Symptom Inhibition. In some cases, positive symptoms may be so strong that inhibitory techniques in isolation may need to be employed. Emphasis, in these instances, is placed on imposing upon the child more normal body postures, helping the child develop a tolerance for them, helping him to maintain them first without and later with auto-excitation, and, finally, helping him to assume the postures without assistance. Examples of this technique follow.

If a child regularly assumes an asymmetrical tonic neck posture in supine or sitting, the clinician should first impose a more normal body posture; second, he should resist the tendency for the child's body parts to return to their former posture; third, he should eventually remove his controlling hands for progressively longer periods of time in order to determine whether and for how long the child can maintain the new posture. After the child shows ability to maintain the posture, he should develop an ability to do so while lateralizing his own head through progressively larger arcs to the right and to the left.

Similar activities may be carried out for other resistant positive symptoms. As another example, if the child cannot maintain a standing posture easily because of exaggerated avoiding responses of the feet (Twitchell, 1965), the child should be placed in an appropriate standing posture, pressure should be applied to the foot or feet, and the withdrawal reaction resisted. If the adaptation procedure is successful, the child should eventually maintain the standing posture without, or with reduced symptoms of the avoiding response.

Body Part Differentiation. Because of the common infantile integration of afferent inflow from the otoliths and neck receptors among the cerebral palsied, and the consequent perseveration of tonic reflexes, specific attention to head and neck differentiation from the rest of the body may be necessary. Essentially, this is accomplished by positioning the individual in an appropriate positive symptom inhibiting posture and then passively lateralizing the head, bending the head in an ear-to-shoulder fashion, as well as ventroflexing and dorsiflexing the head. These head movements are carried out while the clinician resists the emergence of tonic reflexes. The procedures should be executed in all the postures that the child can maintain or be placed in, for example, supine, prone, sitting, and standing. Other parts of the body should be differentiated following similar maneuvers, the goal being to help the child develop the ability to move an arm, leg, forearm, foot, finger, and so on, in isolation. However, since the head leads in all the motor acts engaged in by the human, head and neck differentiation from the rest of the body is of prime importance.

Body Part Adaptation to Sensory Stimuli. To raise the unusually low thresholds in certain cerebral palsied children for the handling of their heads, necks, chests, and so on; to reduce their reactions to muscle elongation; and to eliminate their low crying and laughing thresholds, all of which may impede neurotherapy, efforts should also be made at effecting body part adaptation to various sensory stimuli. Again, this is done essentially by first positioning the individual, and then stimulating him accordingly (wherever possible, with the child's own hands) until the desired tolerance to various stimuli is gradually attained.

Supplementary Tactile-Proprioceptive Techniques

The following tactile-proprioceptive techniques may be used in conjunction with any of the therapy approaches. The procedures may increase or reduce muscle tone; increase general sensory stimulation; excite additional motor units in various muscles; or encourage more normal or correct abnormal sensory feedbacks.

Muscle Tone. Tapping or *stroking* muscle groups may increase or decrease muscle tone depending on the frequency and intensity of the procedure. *Rocking* a child in the arms or on a chair, or *bouncing* the child gently on your knees or on the floor in the seated position, should increase muscle tone and also provide an increased amount of general sensory inflow. *Shaking* a hypertonic limb or organ may reduce muscle tone. By inviting, and then resisting an intended movement, additional motor units may be excited which may cause an increased degree of movement, as well as new movements in a particular body part.

Special Reflexes and Reactions. Placing various body parts in particular positions and then moving the body in various ways should elicit certain normal reflexive movements. For example: placing the child's chin on a horizontal surface, while bringing the body close to a vertical surface should cause the child to flex and raise both arms up to the horizontal surface; placing the child's instep against the edge of a table should cause a stepping-like activity; and holding a child in the air, and then bringing him toward the floor should excite a leg posture appropriate for standing. Hopping reactions or body-supporting leg movements may be elicited by holding the child in an erect position and changing the body's center of gravity by moving the body in various directions. Normal leg extension patterns, as in walking, may be stimulated by holding the child's flexed leg by the foot and tipping the child forward by pulling on his hand (see-saw reaction). Crawling movements may be stimulated by pressing or lifting in the pelvic area while the child is in the prone position. The necessary protective-extensor-thrust of the arms reaction may be stimulated by holding the child in the air at the ankles, or the pelvis, and bringing the child's head toward the ground. The latter four reactions were described in Chapter Two.

Special Postures and Movements. *Variability work,* or placing the child's body parts in various and unusual positions ("pretzeling") and having him work free of them, should reduce muscle tone, effect new sensory inflows, and should contribute to body-image development and body part self-adjustment ability. *Static crawling* describes a procedure where the child is stimulated and guided in using reciprocal movements of the limbs in the crawling position without actually progressing; such guidance ensures more normal sensory feedbacks which may improve actual crawling attempts. Passively moving both arms and hands through various symmetrical but opposite positions (*"antitropic movements"*) produces a desirable type of sensory feedback and may assist in his body-image development. *Sensory fencing* describes a procedure whereby involuntary movements of an involved limb may be reduced by limiting the space in which the limb is allowed to move; the space is delimited by the clinician's hands and the child is supposed to keep from touching either hand with his involved, oscillating part—the procedure very often reveals that the range of oscillation of the child's body part does not always have to be as great. Finally, *"hanging"* activity from a bar, first with both hands and then with either hand, for progressively longer periods of time, may prove useful to some children. The potential benefit from this activity is derived from the experience of total body weight bearing with fully extended upper limbs, and grasp functioning of the hands.

NEUROTHERAPY PROGRAM REQUIREMENTS

The following section of the chapter discusses factors which should be carefully considered by those specialists who may contemplate initiating neurotherapy programs. The successful application of such therapy usually requires not only a good deal of study and practice of the techniques, but also close adherence to certain organizational procedures.

Diagnostic Team

If a neurotherapy program is to be initiated at a clinic, staff considerations are of utmost importance. A lack of true interest, or a lack of thorough preparation (academic and practical), may prevent the program from ever taking form and, consequently, will usually result in an inaccurate assessment of the approach. The presence of at least two neurophysiologically-oriented specialists on the cerebral palsy team is desirable. Their function is to conduct the initial neurodevelopmental analysis, choose candidates, make therapy recommendations and do periodic follow-up examinations.

Therapy Team

Neurotherapy teams made up of one physical therapist, one speech clinician, and one occupational therapist should be formed. Each therapy candidate is assigned to one such team. These therapy teams should confer and discuss general goals as well as particular subgoals; they should periodically perform therapy as a unit.

Criteria for Selection of Candidates

The following criteria, relevant for children as well as their parents, emerged as more or less important as the Newington studies progressed. Experience at other clinics with different staffs, and so on, may render some less important, and possibly result in the addition of criteria not listed.

Candidates. According to Josephy (1949), the cerebral palsies may be subsumed under at least three general etiologic categories.

1. Heredo-degenerative. These are degenerative diseases in which there may be little chance of sustained improvement. The following represent some of the conditions found under this category: Marie's Ataxia, Friedreich's Ataxia, Tuberous Sclerosis, Sturge-Wever-Dimitris Disease, Lipoidoses, Toxoplasmosis, Schilder's Disease, Juvenile General Paresis, and Infantile Paralysis Agitans.

2. *Cranial malformations.* These are congenital and rather static diseases. The following represent some of the conditions found under this category: Hydrocephaly, Microcephaly, Macrocephaly, Defect of Corpus Callosum, Arrhinencephaly, Congenital Cerebellar Ataxia, Hypertelorism, Microgyria, Pachygyria.

3. *Residue of destructive processes group.* The three types of lesions responsible for this group are vascular impairment of blood supply, crushing injury, and inflammatory infections. Two of the conditions found under this category are porencephaly and subdural hematoma.

It is believed that ideal candidates for neurotherapy would represent those cerebral palsies from the third or residue of destructive processes group who are less than severely involved. These are children who began, theoretically, with a normal CNS. However, this is not to imply that severely involved children or children from the other groups as well may not benefit from such therapy.

In addition, candidates should (1) be younger children with little or no history of previous kinds of treatment (the parent's and child's past therapy orientation and philosophy might be so different that the new adjustment would be difficult); (2) reflect demonstrable lower-center CNS reflexes, or positive symptoms, without extremes of muscle tone; (3) show signs of initial favorable responses to positive-symptom inhibiting postures; (4) be children whose weight is within normal limits; (5) be emotionally tractable and motivated toward self-improvement; (6) be children who are able to receive at least daily treatment on an out-patient basis, or better yet, two or three daily treatment periods on an in-patient basis; and (7) be children whose daily life postures can be reduced to appropriate nervous system evolutional levels (e.g., prone or supine, prone supported by forearms, seated) without causing adverse parental or child reactions.

Parents. Parents must be willing and capable of learning therapy techniques. They represent the home carry-over part of the team and are essential. They should be prepared to participate in periodic parent-clinician group therapy sessions.

Records. Records are important for therapy, teaching, and research purposes. Experience thus far has revealed that the following represent records which may be considered as basic for therapy programs and which should be taken at periodic intervals: (1) motion films of active infantile reflexes, highest equilibrium reactions, and of movement from supine to highest level of motor development; (2) notations of abnormal oral and hand reflexes, as well as of the highest types of associated speaking and arm-hand activities; (3) thoracic and abdominal breathing records during vegetative and speech breathing activities; and (4) records of samples of conversational speech and of sustained vowel phonation and of articulatory diadochocinetic rates.

Criteria for Discontinuance of Therapy

Deciding whether or not to continue therapy is always a difficult task; however, after some experience the following four criteria appear to be worth considering when such a decision is to be made: (1) Six-to-nine-month plateau period; (2) Adverse emotional reactions in the child; (3) Irregular attendance; and (4) Lack of home follow-up in regard to therapy and neurophysiological hygiene suggestions.

Discontinuance procedures might include a three- or four-month "clinic holiday" with at least one return to a full therapy program.

APPLICATION OF NEUROEVOLUTIONAL THERAPY PROCEDURES

The results of what is believed to be a first attempt at an organized study of the effects of utilizing neuroevolutional therapy techniques with a group of cerebral palsied children may be found in the phase one and phase two film records made by the author (Mysak, 1960, 1962). A written report on the findings appears below. The description of the subjects will include their: (1) official medical classification as it appeared in their respective records; (2) pretherapy level of general motor development and their level of nervous system evolution; and (3) posttherapy level of general motor development and their level of nervous system evolution. The written reports will contain what was considered only the more important aspects of each child's pretherapy and posttherapy motor and neuroevolutional statuses.

It should also be pointed out that the seven children included in the phase one study were not selected by the investigator but were children who had reached "plateaus" in other therapy programs, or who, for one reason or another, were no longer interesting therapy candidates. Further, the clinicians who worked with the children were learning the therapy approach during the study period. (See purpose number three which follows.)

It will also be noted that a control group in the usual sense of the word was not used in this study. Rather, the study was planned as a subject-oriented one; that is, the children were used as their own controls. Results were evaluated on the basis of whether positive changes took place during the period of therapy, and the extent of such changes as reflected in the pre and posttherapy statuses of each child.

The author considers recent comments made by Jerger in 1964 pertinent, with respect to this type of subject-oriented research. Quotes from his statement follow.

> One of the most exciting developments in contemporary behavioral research is what Arthur Bachrach has called the 'informal theoretical method.' Its principal spokesmen, notably Skinner and Sidman, stress the value of precisely controlled observation on a single subject, experimental manipulation of behavior, and the search for meaningful functional relationships among actual data, in contradistinction to formal theory construction, classical hypothesis testing, and statistical inference about averages.

Relating the statement to research in speech pathology Jerger went on to say

> . . . Is it possible, for example, that the essence of stuttering continues to elude us because of our singular devotion to an experimental design which tests an hypothesis about the difference between the average stutterer and the average non-stutterer?
> . . . Finally, there is a promising area for individual-subject-oriented research in language disorders where the experts repeatedly emphasize that no two aphasics are quite alike, but publish research reports comparing averages for the aphasic group and the control group . . .

In view of the highly variable characteristics of the children that usually make up the cerebral palsied group, subject-oriented research appears to be a most appropriate way of studying these children.

Phase One

The purpose of the initiatory phase of the study conducted at the Newington Hospital for Crippled Children was (1) to ascertain whether Newington's application of neurophysiologic therapy techniques would alter the cerebral palsied child's reflexology in any positive manner; (2) to acquaint concerned staff at the hospital with the therapeutic procedure and rationale; and (3) to serve as a training opportunity for interested clinicians. The following descriptions are of all the seven subjects who appeared in phase one.

Subject 1. This female was diagnosed as a left hemiplegic (acquired at ten months) and was fourteen months old at the beginning of therapy.

Pretherapy testing indicated that she had difficulty in assuming the erect or bipedal posture and that she carried her left arm in a rather typical hemiplegic flexor pattern while walking. A reflexive analysis revealed evidence of the presence of abnormal tonic neck and tonic labyrinthine reflexes. Further, the child had not developed the normal protective-extensor-thrust of the arms reaction. The combination of active tonic neck and tonic labyrinthine reflexes contributed to her arm posture during walking.

After approximately six months of therapy, the child showed a diminution in the strength of the tonic neck and tonic labyrinthine reflexes and the development of a more normal protective-extensor-thrust pattern of the arms. This reflexive change enabled the child to assume the standing position with greater ease and allowed her to carry her arm in a more normal manner during walking.

Subject 2. This male was diagnosed as a child with hypotonia and a mild spastic element and was two years and three months old at the start of therapy.

Pretherapy testing showed that the child had great difficulty in assuming the crawling position as well as difficulty in actual crawling; crawling was marked by a lack of normal limb reciprocation. A reflexive analysis revealed the presence of the abnormal asymmetrical tonic neck reflex, signs of the irregular positive supporting reaction, and the abnormal absence of equilibrium reactions in the supine and sitting positions.

After approximately five months of therapy, there was a weakening of the asymmetrical tonic neck reflex and the positive supporting reaction as well as the development of equilibrium reactions in the supine and sitting positions. The child was then able to assume the crawling position with comparative quickness and manifested an improved crawling capacity characterized by the initiation of a limb reciprocation pattern.

Subject 3. This female was diagnosed as a spastic quadriplegic and was five years and four months old at the beginning of the study.

Pretherapy testing indicated that the child had difficulty in assuming the sitting position from supine, had difficulty in accomplishing the crawling position, and showed deficits in limb reciprocation during crawling. The reflexive analysis revealed a deficient amphibian reaction, absence of the labyrinthine righting reflex acting on the head, and a lack of equilibrium reactions in the supine, sitting, and standing positions.

After approximately nine months of therapy, the amphibian reaction, the labyrinthine righting reflex acting on the head, and equilibrium reactions in supine, sitting, and standing positions were stimulated. In conjunction with these reflexive changes, the child manifested improvement in accomplishing the crawling position and gains in limb reciprocation during crawling.

Subject 4. This female was diagnosed as a spastic quadriplegic and was six years and seven months old at the beginning of the study.

Pretherapy testing revealed that the subject had great difficulty in assuming the crawling position and that she reflected a substantial degree of generalized heightened muscle tone (a pained expression was noted as the child attempted to overcome this abnormal muscle tone during her efforts to move). The reflexive analysis revealed associated reactions in the contralateral arm and leg upon squeezing an object with her left hand; an active Moro reflex; lack of a protective-extensor-thrust pattern of the arms; weakness of the labyrinthine righting reflex acting on the head; and the absence of equilibrium reactions in the sitting and standing positions.

After about nine months of therapy, there was a reduction in the strength of the associated reactions and the Moro reflex, a more normal protective-extensor-thrust pattern of the arms, a stronger labyrinthine righting reflex acting on the head, and the development of equilibrium reactions in sitting and standing. These reflexive changes increased the child's ability to assume the crawling position, and resulted in a substantial improvement in generalized muscle tone and in crawling.

Subject 5. This male was diagnosed as a right spastic hemiplegic and was seven years and nine months old at the beginning of therapy.

The pretherapy evaluation showed a rather typical hemiplegic walking pattern characterized by a flexor posture of the affected arm and a hyperextension tendency of the affected leg when it carried the body weight. A reflexive analysis showed the presence of the asymmetrical tonic neck reflex (active on the side of the involvement), the symmetrical tonic neck reflex, a deficiency in the protective-extensor-thrust of the arms reaction on the right side, and deficits in equilibrium reactions in sitting.

After about nine months of therapy, the strengths of the asymmetrical tonic neck reflex and of the symmetrical tonic neck reflex were reduced, and a more normal protective-extensor-thrust pattern of the arms and more normal equilibrium reactions in sitting were stimulated. In association with these reflexive changes, the child walked with a more normal arm posture and arm swing and, in addition, gains in decreasing the hyperextension pattern of the affected leg during walking were also noted.

Subject 6. This male was diagnosed as a spastic quadriplegic following an undetermined illness when he was seven years and four months old; the child was seven years and eight months old at the beginning of therapy.

Pretherapy testing showed that the child could not assume the standing position unless assisted. During attempts at walking, he showed a strong equinus tendency, unsteadiness, and could only manage a few steps. A reflexive analysis showed the presence of the asymmetrical tonic neck reflex, an almost absent amphibian reaction, a deficient labyrinthine righting reflex acting on the head, and deficient equilibrium reactions in sitting and standing.

After about twelve months of therapy, the asymmetrical tonic neck reflex was weakened, and the amphibian reaction, the labyrinthine righting reflex acting on the head, and equilibrium reactions in sitting and standing were stimulated. This amount of neuroevolutionary progress resulted in a greatly improved walking ability as well as in the development of running activity.

Subject 7. This female was diagnosed as an athetoid quadriplegic and was eleven years and six months old at the beginning of therapy.

Pretherapy testing showed that without assistance the child could not assume the crawling position. A reflexive analysis showed signs of the asymmetrical tonic neck reflex and the absence of the protective-extensor-thrust of the arms reaction and most of the equilibrium reactions.

After about six months of therapy, the asymmetrical tonic neck reflex was weakened, and the protective-extensor-thrust of the arms reaction and some equilibrium reactions were stimulated. This reflexive change allowed the child to assume the crawling position independently, acquire an incipient crawling pattern, and to kneel-stand.

At the close of this initiatory exploration of neurotherapy procedures, it was found that the reflexology of all seven children studied appeared to have been positively influenced. In other words, all the children, to varying degrees, had evolved to higher neuroevolutional levels and hence to higher levels of general motor development.

Phase Two

The following children were included in the second phase of the study. The reasons for conducting phase two were (1) to confirm the unexpected, general positive findings of phase one by working with a different population of cerebral palsied children; and (2) to show how progress may or may not be maintained by including a subject from phase one. Eighteen new children were initially involved in phase two; however, only nine will be discussed here. Even though all the children made at least minimal gains, only those who made the more appreciable gains will be described. Four subjects did not complete the full therapy period because of discharge from the hospital for various reasons not related to the study.

Subject 8. This male was diagnosed as a spastic diplegic and was four years and five months old at the beginning of therapy.

Pretherapy testing revealed that he used an infantile method of assuming the quadrupedal or crawling position; that is, he utilized a complete rotation pattern in order to rise from the supine position. Attempts at kneel-walking were characterized by great difficulty. A reflexive analysis showed the presence of the symmetrical tonic neck and Landau reflexes.

After about thirteen months of therapy, a reduction in the strength of the symmetrical tonic neck reflex and the Landau reflex was accomplished. This reflexive change allowed the child to sit up with an almost symmetrical pattern; to crawl with greater limb reciprocation; to show improved kneel-walking; and to reflect an increased ability to assume the standing position.

Subject 9. This male was diagnosed as a spastic quadriplegic and was nine years and four months old at the start of therapy.

Pretherapy testing showed that he achieved the crawling position by using the complete rotation pattern normally used by children from about ten months up to two or three years. Crawling activity was marked by a deficient limb reciprocation pattern; he also showed difficulty in assuming the kneel-standing position as well as difficulty in kneel-walking. A reflexive analysis revealed the presence of the atypical Landau reflex and absence of equilibrium reactions in the sitting position.

After about twelve months of therapy, the Landau reflex was extinguished and equilibrium reactions in the sitting position were stimulated. This change in reflexive status was accompanied by the development of a mature symmetrical sitting pattern, gains in limb reciprocation during crawling, and increased ability in assuming the kneel-standing position.

Subject 10. This male was diagnosed as a spastic diplegic and was three years and five months old at the beginning of therapy.

Pretherapy testing indicated that the child needed assistance from the tester in order to accomplish the standing position. Also, walking was characterized by a swaying motion. Reflexive testing revealed signs of the asymmetrical and symmetrical tonic neck reflexes.

After about twelve months of therapy, the infantile reflexes were substantially weakened. This situation resulted in the child's being able to assume the standing position without assistance and also in a much-improved walking pattern.

Subject 11. This male was diagnosed as a spastic triplegic and was five years and two months old at the start of therapy.

Pretherapy testing indicated that the child had difficulty in accomplishing the crawling position and that body progression was achieved with a "two-point" crawling pattern. A reflexive analysis revealed that, among other reflexive deficits, the child did not show an amphibian reaction.

After about twelve months of therapy, motor improvement was manifested by an increased ability in achieving the quadrupedal position, better crawling, and the ability to kneel-stand.

Subject 12. This male was diagnosed as a spastic quadriplegic and was six years and ten months old at the start of therapy.

Pretherapy testing showed that the child had difficulty in assuming the standing position, showed substantial insecurity in that position, and manifested a poor limb reciprocation pattern during walking. The reflexive analysis showed evidence of the symmetrical tonic neck reflex during walking and deficient hopping reactions.

Following about thirteen months of therapy, the symmetrical tonic neck reflex during walking was almost completely eliminated and active hopping reactions were stimulated. This reflexive change resulted in the child's being able to assume the standing position with greater ease and balance and to show an improved walking pattern.

Subject 13. This female was diagnosed as a case of cerebral atrophy with cerebral-palsy-like symptoms and was two years and five months old at the start of therapy.

Pretherapy testing indicated that the child had to use a complete rotation pattern in order to achieve the quadrupedal position from the supine. Body progression was accomplished by a "two-point" crawling pattern. The reflexive analysis revealed the presence of the symmetrical tonic neck reflex; in addition, there was a lack of equilibrium reactions in the sitting position.

After about twelve months of therapy, the symmetrical tonic neck reflex was noticeably weakened and equilibrium reactions in the sitting position were stimulated. In conjunction with this reflexive evolution, the child was able to achieve the quadrupedal position more easily, crawled in a more normal fashion, and was able to kneel-stand.

Subject 14. This female was diagnosed as a spastic quadriplegic and was ten years and nine months old at the beginning of the study.

Pretherapy testing showed that she experienced substantial difficulty both in assuming the quadrupedal position and in crawling; she also exhibited a definite amount of lordosis during kneel-standing and kneel-walking activities. The reflexive analysis showed the presence of the asymmetrical tonic neck reflex and weak equilibrium reactions in the sitting position.

After about twelve months of therapy, the asymmetrical tonic neck reflex was weakened and equilibrium reactions in sitting were well developed. In conjunction with this reflexive change, the child achieved the quadrupedal position with comparative ease; showed an improved crawling pattern; accomplished kneel-standing with ease; and kneel-walked with increased ability. In addition, the last two activities were done with a substantial reduction in the amount of associated lordosis.

Subject 15. This female was diagnosed as a mixed spastic and athetoid type and was six years and five months old at the beginning of therapy.

Pretherapy testing showed that the child had a great deal of difficulty in her attempts at achieving the quadrupedal position; a great amount of associated involuntary movement was also observable. The reflexive analysis showed the presence of the asymmetrical tonic neck reflex, a lack of the amphibian reaction, and the lack of equilibrium reactions in the sitting position.

After about twelve months of therapy, the strength of the asymmetrical tonic neck reflex was greatly reduced and the amphibian reaction and equilibrium reactions in sitting were stimulated. This reflexive change resulted in an increased ability to accomplish the quadrupedal position. An obvious lessening of involuntary movements was also noted.

Subject 7 (phase one). As previously stated, a child from phase one of the study was included in phase two in order to determine whether continued progress might be obtained if neurotherapy were continued over a substantial period of time.

At the beginning of the phase one therapy period the child could not assume the quadrupedal position unless assisted; however, after six months (end of phase one) she was able to achieve the quadrupedal position independently, showed some crawling behavior, and was able to kneel-stand. After a total of three years of therapy (end of phase two), she was able to move into the quadrupedal position with greater ease; crawl better; kneel-stand with increased control and balance; kneel-walk in an improved manner; maintain standing balance; and, finally, even to take her first steps in walking.

Conclusions

The data from both phase one and two of the study indicate that there is value in applying Jacksonian concepts in the evaluation of children with cerebral palsy; that is, in determining the child's level of CNS arrestment, retardation, or dissolution with its accompanying positive symptoms. The findings also reveal that positive symptoms apparently do prevent the child from manifesting his full neuroevolutional potential. It was shown further, that via special techniques, these positive symptoms may be weakened, higher-order sensorimotor integration stimulated, and, consequently, a higher neuroevolutional level achieved.

Before concluding this section of the chapter additional data which should prove of value to occupational therapists and teachers concerned with the education of the child with cerebral palsy will be presented.

NEUROEVOLUTION OF ARM-HAND ACTIVITY

The following discussion concentrates on the head-arm-hand relationship which is so important in occupational therapy (Mysak and Fiorentino, 1961); however, other important aspects of occupational therapy for the cerebral palsied should of course be included in the therapy program. Appendix B contains a sample form that may be used in the initial examination of head-arm-hand activities.

Arm-Hand Positive-Symptom Inhibiting Postures

Specific arm-hand stimulation should begin only after the child can respond to inhibiting postures which are conducive to arm-hand activities; for example, in prone while resting on the forearms, or sitting.

Limb Differentiation

Basic arm-hand activities should be possible without eliciting associated reflexes which may cause movements or changes in muscle tonus in different parts of the body. In other words, the therapist should differentiate (1) the head and dominant arm from the rest of the body; (2) the arm from the head; (3) the upper arm from the forearm; (4) the wrist from the forearm; and (5) the fingers from the wrist.

As an illustration of limb differentiation, suppose that as an individual bends his head just before working at a table he excites neck proprioceptors which elicit the abnormal symmetrical tonic neck reflex. This reflex may cause an increase in arm flexor tone and an increase in leg extensor tone, both of which make eye-arm-hand activities more difficult. This situation may be counteracted by first placing the individual in a sitting inhibiting posture; then, while maintaining a leg flexor and arm extensor pattern, exciting neck proprioceptors by raising and lowering the head. Resisting the abnormal arm and leg movements during the head activity may eventually weaken the symmetrical tonic neck reflex and hence contribute to the differentiation of the head and arm from the rest of the body.

Limb Adaptation to Sensory Stimuli

Twitchell (1958a) has reported that primitive hand movements may be seen in cases of brain lesion. The spastic hand as it reaches to grasp may show a finger extension-abduction pattern with a concomitant extension of the wrist. Similar reactions may be evoked by tactile stimulation of parts of the hand. This type of reaction has been described as the avoiding response because of its characteristics. Grasping under these circumstances is at best very difficult and at worst impossible. The athetotic hand according to Twitchell (1958b) may show an extension-abduction pattern when the dorsum of the hand is stimulated and a flexion-adduction pattern (grasp reflex) when the medial border of the palm is stimulated. The athetotic hand represents therefore, a conflict between the grasp reflex and the avoiding response of the hand.

In the case of the spastic hand, the goal in therapy would be to desensitize the avoiding response and stimulate grasping activity. This goal may be achieved by (1) applying pressure (with the thumb) to the palm of the child's hand, then slowly shifting the pressure in the direction of the child's fingertips, thus stimulating finger flexion; or (2) holding the child's fingers in a grasp position while stimulating the dorsum of his hand and physically preventing the emergence of the avoiding response of the hand.

Facilitation of Automatic Hand Movements

Automatic hand movements follow a particular maturational sequence and should be facilitated in accordance with the child's ·level of hand movement maturation. Appendix A outlines hand-movement maturation through the first eighteen months as follows: At about one month: grasp reflex and hand to mouth; two months: grasp in pronation; three months: pulls, hands are loose; four months: placing response of upper limb and clutching; five months: scratches, rakes (ulnar); seven months: slaps, scratches, rakes (whole); eight months: radial raking, scissor grasp; ten months: hitting, pushing, waves, shakes, clasps, pincer grasp; twelve to eighteen months: release. Appropriate movements may be facilitated by exposing the hand to materials, textures, and objects which tend to stimulate desired movements such as raking (e.g., sand), shaking (e.g., rattle), and so on.

Refined Hand Movements

Ideally, only after the child can assume a good sitting inhibiting posture and has had primitive hand reflexes desensitized, has experienced differentiation of the head and arm, and so on, and has had basic hand movements facilitated, should specific refined motor tasks be taught. Therefore, if, for example, a child is to be allowed pencil work, basic hand activities such as hitting, pushing, waving, shaking, and pincer grasp and release should, ideally, have first been accomplished.

Related to the goals of occupational therapy is Jackson's statement: ". . . what on the lowest level are centres for simple reflex actions of eyes and hands are evolved in the highest centres into the physical bases of visual and tactual ideas," (8, p. 91).

Report of a Case Study

For the purpose of objectifying the therapeutic possibilities of the above-described approach, a case report will be presented. This interesting report appeared in the article cited at the beginning of this discussion of arm-hand stimulation.

A fifteen year old hemiplegic female received a

modified neurophysiological approach to treatment which consisted of isolated techniques for the upper extremities only. (Since this girl was in a cast and usually in a wheel chair, the techniques applied were limited accordingly.) Testing for primitive reflexes revealed the presence of strong asymmetrical and symmetrical tonic neck reflexes as well as associated reactions. Because of this situation no active extension of the wrist and fingers or supination was possible. There was also a severe lack of sensation throughout the left extremity . . . the following progress was noted over a seven-month period:

(1) Reduction in abnormal muscle tone was apparent and showed good carry-over from one treatment session to another.

(2) Asymmetrical and symmetrical tonic neck reflexes were substantially weakened; however, the influence of these reflexes continued to reflect itself in the wrist and fingers to varying degrees.

(3) Associated reactions of the left upper extremity had diminished markedly.

(4) Equilibrium and protective reactions could be elicited with no primitive flexion pattern of the elbow occurring so that the patient now walked with a more normal carriage of the arm.

(5) Patient could initiate supination and therapist was able to supinate passively to full range with little difficulty.

(6) An interesting change in sensory capacity was observed. Following is a comparison made between the pretherapy sensory test and the one done at the end of three months of treatment:

SENSORY CAPACITY	PRETHERAPY (*Percentage*)	POSTTHERAPY (*Percentage*)
Response to light touch and pressure	50	80
Response to temperature change	25	100
Stereognosis:		
Rough	50	100
Smooth	50	100
Soft	0	50
Hard	0	50
Flat	100	100
Round, square	0	25
Big, little, long, short	0	0
Position sense:		
Wrist	0	75
Fingers	0	0

FACILITATION OF SENSORY-PERCEPTUAL-
SYMBOLIC ACTIVITY

As for classroom work, it is believed that cerebral palsied children should be in learning postures appropriate to their neuromaturational level. In this regard, a good many children should not be in their usual seated positions if they do not possess the head, neck, and thoracic balance necessary for self-supporting sitting behavior. Under these adverse circumstances, abnormal postures, movements, and muscle tone are likely to increase with concomitant distortion of sensory-perceptual feedbacks. Prone postures on either mats or tables may be far more conducive to learning, if these represent the child's level of neuroevolution.

In addition, the classroom teacher, or better yet a therapist-assistant, should periodically place the children into inhibiting postures during the class time. It would be ideal if, for the greater part of their daily classroom periods, the children could experience states of near normal muscle tone.

Two other factors with respect to learning processes in the cerebral palsied should be considered by the classroom teacher. First, to counteract the tendency for many of these children to suffer "experiential deprivation" every effort should be made to reify all matters being taught. This means the use in teaching of actual objects rather than pictures whenever possible, and as much environmental exploration and field work as possible. In short, every effort should be made to associate teaching of anything with the actual related sights, sounds, touches, tastes, and smells.

The second factor is related to recent reports by Birch (1962, 1963, 1964) of intersensory development. Intersensory development refers to that development whereby sensory information received from one modality is modified by the simultaneous activity of other sense organs. The related concept of sensory modality dominance refers to the tendency for distance receptors such as audition and vision to become progressively more important in conveying information to the individual than the near and internal receptors which are important in early childhood. Increased intersensory collaboration and sensory modality dominance appear to emerge as a function of maturation; however, data are indicating that such synesthesia and sensory dominance may be delayed or distorted in the cerebral palsied.

It would be well if teachers considered the use of synesthetic experiences and ways of facilitating the development of sensory dominance when planning their lessons.

In summary, this rather long chapter included a discussion of the rationale for neurotherapy, neurophysiological considerations in developing therapy procedures, three general types of neurotherapy programs, requirements for developing neurotherapy programs, the results of a two-part study of the actual application of neurotherapy, and, finally, a discussion of the application of neuroevolutional concepts to head-arm-hand activity and to sensory-perceptual-symbolic activity.

Part Two of the book is devoted to the application of neuroevolutional concepts to the origins of speech in man, and to speech development, speech disorder, and speech therapy in cerebral palsy.

REFERENCES

Birch, H. G. "Dyslexia and the Maturation of the Visual Function." John Money (Ed.), *Reading Disability*, Baltimore: The Johns Hopkins Press, 1962.

Birch, H. G. and Lefford, A. "Intersensory development in children," *The Society for Research in Child Development Monogr.*, 1963.

Birch, H. G. and Lefford, A. "Two Strategies for Studying Perception in Brain-Damaged Children." Herbert G. Birch (Ed.), *Brain Damage in Children: The Biological and Social Aspects*, Baltimore: Williams and Wilkins Co., 1964.

Jackson, J. H. "Evolution and Dissolution of the Nervous System" in James Taylor (Ed.), *Selected Writings of John Hughlings Jackson*. Vol. 2. New York: Basic Books, Inc., 1958.

Jerger, J. "Viewpoint: Subject oriented research," *J. Speech Hearing Res.*, 7 (1964), 207–208.

Josephy, H. "The brain in cerebral palsy, a neuropathological review," *Nerv. Child*, 8 (1949), 152–159.

Magnus, R. *Koerperstellung*. Berlin: Springer, 1924.

Mysak, E. D. "Dysarthria and oropharyngeal reflexology: a review," *J. Speech Hearing Dis.*, 28 (1963), 252–260.

Mysak, E. D. Pilot Study Films of a Neurophysiological Approach to Cerebral Palsy Habilitation: Part Two. Film released by the Newington Hospital for Crippled Children, Newington, Connecticut, November, 1962.

Mysak, E. D. Pilot Study Films of a Neurophysiological Approach to Cerebral Palsy Habilitation. Film released by the Newington Hospital for Crippled Children, Newington, Connecticut, June, 1960.

Mysak, E. D. "Significance of neurophysiological orientation to cerebral palsy habilitation," *J. Speech Hearing Dis.*, 24 (1959), 221–230.

Mysak, E. D. and Fiorentino, M. R. "Neurophysiological considerations in occupational therapy for the cerebral palsy," *Amer. J. Occup. Ther.*, 15 (1961), 112–117.

Russell, W. R. "The physiology of memory." *Proc. Roy. Soc. Med.*, 51 (1958), 9–14.

Twitchell, T. E. "The grasping deficit in infantile spastic hemiparesis," *Neurology*, 8 (1958), 13–21.

Twitchell, T. E. "Neurophysiological aspects of congenital bilateral athetosis," *Program. Amer. Acad. Neurol.*, 10 (1958), 22.

Twitchell, T. E. "Variations and abnormalities of motor development," *J. Amer. Phys. Ther. Assoc.*, 45 (1965), 424–430.

Neurogenesis of the Speech System, Neurological Speech Disorder, and Neurospeech Therapy

Neuroevolution of Speech

Part Two of this book consists of two chapters. Chapter Four is concerned with certain neuroevolutional theories of speech and Chapter Five is concerned with the cerebral palsy speech syndrome and with neurospeech therapy procedures.

It is obvious to those interested in speech development that there is a relationship between adequate speech behavior and a certain degree of neuroevolution of the speech system. The study of this relationship by speech specialists is especially important if they are to work effectively with the respiratory-phonatory-articulatory complexes found among the cerebral palsied. The following section of this chapter attempts to outline the neuroevolution of the speech system.

BIPEDAL EVOLUTION AND SPEECH

It would be well if the speech pathologist reminded himself of the connection between the advent of propositional speech and human, bipedal neurophysiological evolution; that is, the connection between efficient speech production and bipedal head, neck, and trunk balance and a bipedal form of respiratory activity (i.e., breathing with the thorax in an erect position). Further, the speech specialist should be aware of the child's general level of CNS evolution if he is to understand more fully human speech development, or, in the case of many cerebral palsied children, if he is to understand better the arrestment or retardation of such development.

ORONEUROMOTOR EVOLUTION AND SPEECH

Another phenomenon which is usually concurrent with bipedal maturation, and which influences speech proficiency, is the development and extinction of certain infantile oroneuromotor activity. It is interesting to note that standard literature in speech pathology contains little in the way of any organized material in what would appear to be a most appropriate area of study, that is, oroneuromotor maturation. Speech-related reflexology will be discussed in this portion of the chapter under three headings. It should be indicated that categorizing the phenomena under the various headings was not always simple and clear and, in fact, in some instances was done on a rather arbitrary basis. It is hoped that the information provided, relative to the ascending development of speech-related reflexology, will not only help the specialist in understanding speech system neuroevolution but will also help him in diagnosing and planning therapy for neurological speech disorders. Some of the information offered below has already been presented by the author in two previous publications (Mysak, 1963, 1965).

Many of the reflexes and reactions discussed under the headings of protective and withdrawal, vegetative, and emotional responses vary in terms of ease, place, and time of elicitation. Time of extinction of these infantile responses also varies from child to child and, therefore, exact information on when some of these reflexes are inhibited cannot be offered. However, it could be stated that, in general, those reflexes which are associated with infantile feeding behavior disappear before or by approximately one year of age. It should also be noted that increased complexity and inconsistency of response distinguishes "reaction" from "reflex."

Protective Reflexes and Withdrawal Reactions

The heading of protective reflexes and withdrawal reactions signifies that the movements described under this category are considered to be designed in some way to protect the organism.

Laryngeal or Glottic Closing Reflex. Laryngeal-closing reflex activity is present during aquatic fetal life. It is interesting that Schwartz (1961) has cited excessive rehearsal of this reflex as a possible cause of infantile voice difficulty, that is, as a cause of congenital laryngeal stridor. Laryngeal closure during swallowing is, of course, a most important reflexive activity for air-breathing organisms and Schwartz believes that prenatal practice of this pattern contributes to its establishment. It was indicated that adults experience this glottic closing reflex during a sudden descent (elevator, plane entering an air pocket), when suddenly splashed with cold water, or when first entering cold water for a swim. Schwartz (1961) described the phenomenon as ". . . the glottis reacting as if it recalled menacing stimuli of an earlier period (immersion reflex)."

Cephalic Reactions. Irregular movements of the head in infants may be elicited by stimulation of the face. Auriculocephalic and naso-cephalic reactions are elicited, respectively, by rubbing the lobe of the ear or tickling the nostril. Such stimulation causes the head to rotate to the opposite side. These withdrawal type reactions have been identified by André-Thomas, *et al.* (1960, p. 5) during the neonatal period.

Coughing and sneezing reflexes may also be listed under the category of protective reflexes and withdrawal reactions.

Vegetative Reflexes

The reflexes and reactions described here are associated with infantile feeding and respiratory behavior.

Respiration. In infancy, lung expansion is accomplished principally by the lowering of the diaphragm. Hence, in the infant, abdominal respiratory movements predominate while thoracic respiratory movements are minimal. Also breathing is shallow and breaths per minute (bpm) are high. Ranges and mean values of respirations per minute given by various investigators have been reported by Peiper (1963, p. 311). For example, up to about the first month the range is from about 22 to 72 bpm; from about the first to the sixth month the range is from 21 to 58 bpm; from about six months to two years the range is from approximately 25 to 45 bpm; from two to five years the range is from 21 to 40 bpm; and from five to ten years the range is from 15 to 31 bpm.

After the sixth month, the predominantly diaphragmatic respiration is gradually replaced by a mixed respiration in which both the diaphragm and thorax participate—breathing is also deeper and slower by the sixth month.

Diaphragmatic breathing is considered to be phylogenetically older than thoracic respiration.

Cardinal Points Reaction. Lightly stroking outwards at the angle of the mouth causes the lowering of the respective half of the lower lip; if the tester's finger is moved away but kept in contact with the cheek, the tongue will move toward the stimulus and the head will follow it. Stimulating the middle of the upper and lower lips will cause lip and tongue raising or depression, respectively; if the tester's finger continues to move upwards, or downwards toward the chin the head will extend, or the mouth open and the head flex, respectively (André-Thomas, *et al.*, 1960, p. 15). Rooting reflex is another way of identifying the cardinal points reaction. In his discussion of rooting reflexes Prechtl (1958) speaks specifically of side-to-side and directed head-turning phases. The first phase, which lasts from birth to about three weeks, is characterized by side-to-side head turning which decreases in extent as the head is gradually directed toward the stimulus. After about three weeks, a single well-guided movement of the head, which brings it in contact with the touch stimulus, or the directed head-turning reflex emerges. Gentle tapping or stroking of the cheek, perioral skin, or lips constitutes the adequate stimulus. Time of disappearance of the directed head-turning reflex varies and it is not unusual to observe it at the age of one year.

Hand-Mouth Reflexes. There are at least two hand-mouth coordination reflexes which can be found in the newborn and which may be explained on a phyletic basis—the palmar-mental reflex and the palmar-mandibular reflex (Peiper, 1963, p. 116, pp. 416–417). The palmar-mental reflex is elicited by scratching the thenar eminence. Simultaneous contraction of the chin muscles which lifts the chin up constitutes the response pattern. The reflex has been reported in newborn infants, in infants up to the last months of the first year, and occasionally in children between six to twelve years.

The palmar-mandibular reflex, or Babkin's reflex, can be elicited by applying pressure to the palms of both hands. Mouth-opening, closing of eyes, and head ventroflexion constitutes the response pattern. The response weakens during the first month and usually disappears by the third month.

The phyletic heritage of these patterns is related to manner of food intake. The lower form of food intake (used, e.g., by fish, amphibians, reptiles) is by direct mouth seizure and oral manipulation. This lower form of food intake is reflected by the human infant during the time he is utilizing the rooting-feeding pattern. The higher form of intake involves first grasping the food with the limbs and then bringing it to the mouth. This manner of food intake is used by the older infant as well as by animals such as the squirrel and monkey.

In cases of neuropathology in children and adults, these infantile hand-mouth reflexes may be retained or may re-appear as positive symptoms.

Mouth-Opening Reflex. At about four months, a visual stimulus such as a breast, bottle or finger may effect reflexive mouth-opening (Mysak, 1959).

Lip Reflex or Mouth Phenomena. Tapping near the angle of the mouth evokes involuntary movements of the lips in addition to eventual lip closure and pouting activity as in preparation for suckling (Thomson, 1903). Time of disappearance fluctuates greatly; it has been elicited in some normal children up to twelve years when they were in a drowsy or sleepy state.

Biting Reflex. In response to a stimulus object placed between the gums, mouth-closure and holding behavior may be noticed. The reflex can usually be inhibited by approximately four months (Mysak, 1959).

⤳*Suckling Reflex.* Placing the finger or nipple in contact with the lips, front of tongue, gums, or hard palate elicits a suckling response. Gentle movement of the stimulus object usually facilitates the activity. Suckling constitutes a forward, upward, and backward movement of the tongue. Thus, it is differentiated from what is commonly called sucking which is basically a holding of the stimulus object between the lips while creating negative pressure within the mouth. The suckling reflex usually can be inhibited from about four months (Mysak, 1959) up to the first year; however, it has been elicited in drowsy, older children by gentle stroking of the lips.

⤳*Chewing Reflex.* At about seven months reflexive chewing may be excited by stimulating the gum or teeth with a finger or a biscuit (Illingworth, 1962, p. 25).

It should be of interest and of value to note that Hooker (1952) found infantile cranio-oropharyngeal patterns similar to the rooting, lip, mouth-opening, biting, suckling, and the cephalic motor patterns described here in human fetuses between 7.5 and 26 weeks menstrual age (number of weeks since onset of last menstrual period before conception). The patterns were described as reflexive, as appearing in an orderly progression with fetal development, and as resulting from excitation of the trigeminal nerve.

On the basis of clinical observation, conditions of abnormal release or retention of many of the reflexes and reactions described is believed to cause, directly or indirectly and to varying degrees, interference with articulatory behavior. More specifically, when attempted articulatory movements also elicit infantile reflexes which, for example, cause involuntary jaw deviation, lip movement, mouth-opening, and tongue protrusion, it may be appreciated that these extraneous movements may make adequate articulation more difficult.

In contrast to the infantile feeding reactions and reflexes described above, which disappear before or by approximately one year of age, the following reflexes are normally present throughout life. They are presented because they represent responses which, in addition to their diagnostic pertinence (some may be lost or weakened in cases of dysarthria), may also have value when used in remedial procedures. The latter point will be elaborated upon in the next chapter.

⤳*Swallowing Reflex.* Stimulation of the palate, fauces, posterior pharyngeal wall, or back of the tongue will cause swallowing activity (Miller, Sherrington, 1915). In addition, coughing, sneezing, and hiccoughing are usually followed by swallowing. Swallowing also precedes or follows suckling activity. In the neonatal period, swallowing is usually preceded by mouth-opening and protrusion and subsequent retraction of the tongue, or preceded by the suckling reflex. A change in this pattern may be observed at about twelve weeks; at this time, the tongue may not protrude as the mouth is opened. However, in some normal infants the tongue protrusion pattern may be retained for as yet undetermined reasons. Swallowing difficulty (dysphagia) is usually encountered in cases of spastic dysarthria (Brain, 1955, p. 94).

Pharyngeal Reflex. In response to a touch upon the posterior pharyngeal wall, contraction of the constrictor muscles of the pharynx may be observed (Brain, 1955, p. 42). Stimulation of the fauces may also elicit the pharyngeal or gag reflex. This reflex may be weakened in certain cases of dysarthria (Brain, 1955, pp. 42, 94).

Palatal Reflex. This reflex consists of velar elevation in response to touch (Brain, 1955, p. 42). It may also be affected in certain cases of dysarthria (Brain, 1955, p. 42).

Yawning, that is, deep involuntary inspiration with the mouth open, may also be listed under this category of reflexes.

Emotional Reflexes

Those reflexes which are usually associated with different types of affect, or those reactions which automatically accompany feelings of pleasantness or unpleasantness elicited by various external or internal stimuli, may be referred to as emotional reflexes.

Laughter Reflex. Tickling may elicit uncontrollable laughter in infants. Illingworth (1962, p. 24) reports laughing behavior in infants at about sixteen weeks.

Smiling Reflex. Reflexive smiling in response to the maternal voice may be demonstrated at about four to six weeks (Illingworth, 1962, p. 25). The smiling reflex may also be evoked by auditory, visual, or movement stimuli.

Sobbing and sighing activities may also be listed under this category. All these emotional reflexes, of course, have communicative value for adults.

Knowledge of the above reflexes and reactions should first of all allow the diagnostician to determine their presence or absence in any given case of dysarthria, and secondly help him to assess the possible contribution of the phenomena to the total articulatory problem. It may be found that various extraneous movements, including articulatory attempts themselves, may trigger many of these reflexes.

It might also be pointed out at this time that most of the reflexes associated with infantile feeding behavior are inhibited by the time the normal child utters two- or three-word sentences. In other words, articulatory movements, which require higher integrated motor activity, are apparently more adequately performed when infantile oral reflex behavior has been inhibited. Recognition of this normal process of oral reflexive maturation should make it easier to understand why retained or released infantile oral reflexes may hinder articulatory activity and why they consequently may compound certain cases of dysarthria.

Awareness of these responses may also aid the clinician in detecting and evaluating the influence of persisting infantile oral reflexes in many cases of nonparalytic articulatory problems which may now be considered as functional or idiopathic.

RELATIONSHIP OF ORONEUROMOTOR EVOLUTION TO ARTICULATORY BEHAVIOR

A discussion of how infantile oroneuromotor activity may contribute to articulatory disorders appears in Chapter Five; however, it might be interesting at this time to hypothesize about the possible relationships between infantile oropharyngeal reflexology and speech behavior in general.

Many of the infantile oral reflexes and reactions described may be viewed as background movement patterns ('rehearsal phenomena') which contribute to the more complex movement patterns needed for prelinguistic phonatory and articulatory behavior. In this vein, Meader (1940) spoke of articulatory movements as modified vegetative reflexes. She also recommended the build-up of vegetative reflexes such as swallowing, sucking, and chewing in therapy for hyphoid speech.

Associations with respect to the concept of rehearsal phenomena and speech behavior follow: (1) Respiratory activities involved in coughing, sobbing, sighing, yawning, and laughing may be considered as making a contribution to the development of the respiratory movements needed in speech production; some of these phenomena also possess communicative value (Travis, 1931, p. 7). (2) The laryngeal or glottic closing reflex may be viewed as a precursory movement to the laryngeal activity required for human voice production. (3) Rooting reflex activity may be seen as an initial and primitive inter-communication act between the nursing mother and her child; that is, it may be seen as a preliminary form of face-to-face behavior which later serves as a base for speaker-listener interaction. It should also be mentioned that rooting-feeding activity by the infant is frequently accompanied by a good deal of maternal talking. (4) Lip reflex activity including pouting and closure sequences may be viewed as preliminary movements for vowel, bilabial, and labiodental sound production. (5) Mouth-opening activity could represent the background movements required for the production of sounds requiring varying degrees of mandibular extension and flexion. (6) Biting, suckling, swallowing, and chewing patterns may be seen as forerunner activities for those articulatory patterns required for linguadental, lingua-alveolar, linguapalatal and lingua-velar speech sounds. (7) Finally, muscle patterns used in suckling, swallowing, pharyngeal, palatal, and yawning reflexes may be viewed as antecedent activity which contributes to the velopharyngeal closure patterns needed during speech production.

CORTICALIZATION, DOMINANCE AND SPEECH

A good deal has been written lately on the relationship between the evolution of the cortex, with reference to the increase in size of certain cortical areas and hemispheral dominance, and speech development. This is a discussion of these relationships based on ideas and observations of various authorities.

Uncommitted Cortex

Penfield's contribution to the understanding of speech via his work on the surgical treatment of epilepsy (Penfield and Roberts, 1959) should be familiar to all individuals interested in speech theory. Material of particular pertinence to this portion of the chapter may be found in a recent chapter by Penfield (1966) in which he discusses the concept of the uncommitted cortex.

Penfield (1966, pp. 219–220) stated, ". . . Man's brain is remarkable among mammals because of the greatly increased volume of cerebral cortex that covers it with deeply folded convolutions." He continues, "Unlike the cortex of the rat, which is completely motor or sensory except for a small undefined area, most of the human cortex is neither sensory in function nor motor." Penfield then presents data illustrating the successively greater increase in the proportion of uncommitted cortex as compared with the sensory and motor cerebral cortex in the brains of the rat, ground shrew, tree shrew, tarsius, chimpanzee, and finally man. According to Penfield, ". . . The temporal and parietal lobes have made their appearance in man as an outbudding from the thalamus which seems to push the visual sensory cortex back and away from the somatic sensory and the auditory sensory."

He goes on to say that the motor and sensory areas of man's cortex are committed as to function, but that this is not the case with respect to the new cortex between the auditory and the visual areas. The organizational and functional connections of the new cortex are established during the first decade of life. The new cortex is devoted to speech in the major hemisphere (usually left) and to perception in the minor hemisphere.

Penfield supports his view by presenting information collected from conscious patients who were undergoing brain surgery. He stated that when electrical current was applied to the speech cortex (major hemisphere) an immediate interference (aphasia-like) with the speech mechanism was observed; however, no such occurrence was observed when electrical stimulation was applied to the corresponding area in the minor hemisphere. Instead, stimulation in the minor hemisphere may be found to result in two types of phenomena.

One type of response is manifested by the patient reporting that ". . . what he sees and hears seems suddenly familiar, or strange, or frightening, or coming closer, or going away, etc." (Penfield, 1966, p. 221). Another type of response is characterized by the patient's sudden ". . . awareness of some previous experience." That is, he experiences a sudden "flashback."

Penfield reported that similar "psychical responses" can be elicited by electrical stimulation ". . . of the temporal cortex that lies farther forward on the nondominant side and on the dominant side as well. Thus, except for the speech area and the audiosensory area, the cortex that covers the superior and lateral surfaces of the temporal lobe on both sides may be taken as a functional unit" (Penfield, 1966, p. 221). Since Penfield considers the function of this unit to be interpretive in nature, the area responsible for such responses has been named the "interpretive cortex."

Concepts which may be drawn from Penfield's statements and which have pertinence to the discussion of the neuroevolution of speech are first, the emergence of an uncommitted cortex in man, and second, the emergence of the speech cortex in the uncommitted cortex of the dominant hemisphere. Also pertinent to our discussion is Penfield's belief that the speech cortex is composed of a major speech area (Werniche's area) and two minor speech areas (Broca's area and the supplementary motor area); and that destruction of the major speech area results in loss of speech, but that if the damage occurs before the age of ten or twelve the homologous area on the nondominant side may develop into a speech area within the period of a year or more. Damage to this homologous area in the nondominant hemisphere in the adult causes problems in the awareness of body scheme and of spatial relationships.

Speech Dominance

Additional ideas with respect to cerebral dominance and speech were recently offered by Roberts (1966).

After a very brief review of the history of theories on the relationships among speech function, cerebral dominance, and handedness,

Roberts (1966, p. 18) sums up by saying that, "Handedness is a form of behavior in a particular individual. It may be influenced by psychological abnormalities, heredity, environment, brain damage, and perhaps other factors." Of pertinence to our discussion of the neuroevolution of speech is Roberts' statement that, regardless of handedness, the left hemisphere is usually dominant for speech purposes except in those cases where individuals have suffered damage to the left cerebral hemisphere at an early age.

Roberts states further that he feels ". . . the most important thing man inherits is a left cerebral hemisphere dominant for speech." He also believes it possible ". . . that right-handedness may have developed secondarily to speech dominance." Conversely, if, in fact, the right hemipshere is dominant for speech, the chances are the individual will be left-handed.

A brief review of Roberts' findings, including a discussion of effects of lesions and of electrical stimulation of the brain, should also make a contribution to the purpose of this chapter. Roberts describes the following lesions which specifically affect speech and language. (1) Bilateral lesions in the region of the inferior Rolandic fissure cause symptoms of pseudobulbar palsy and anarthria or dysarthria. (2) Lesions in the supplementary motor area of Penfield result in aphasia and difficulty in producing rapidly alternating movements, especially in the opposite foot; also, similar difficulty may be experienced in oral activities. However, the entire supplementary motor area may be excised without permanent aphasia. (3) Lesions in the region of the posterior part of the second frontal convolution cause aphasia associated with writing difficulties, but is transient. (4) Lesions in the region of the posterior part of the third frontal convolution, or Broca's area, cause an aphasia which will also resolve itself. (5) "The most pronounced and prolonged disturbances in speech occur with lesions of the posterior speech area—the posterior temporal, inferior parietal, and anterior occipital region. The more anterior the lesion, the more the auditory aspects of speech are involved, and the more posterior the lesion, the more the visual aspects are effected." (Roberts, 1966, p. 21.)

Roberts (1966, pp. 21–22) offered the following information with respect to the effects on speech of electrically stimulating various parts of the cerebral cortex. He reports on both positive and negative effects of such stimulation. (1) Positive effects, either continuous or intermittent vowel-like vocalization—sometimes with consonant components, have been produced by stimulation of both primary and supplementary motor areas of both hemispheres. (2) Negative effects, that is, arrest of speech, hesitation, slurring, and repetition of words or syllables have been observed when the motor areas of both hemispheres have been stimulated. Such negative effects also occurred when the dominant Broca's and temporoparietal regions were stimulated. Roberts considers that these effects are related to interference with either motor or speech systems. Confusion during counting, naming difficulty with retained ability to speak, and naming difficulty with or without perseveration, are other negative symptoms reported by Roberts and have been elicited from the dominant Broca's, supplementary motor, and temporoparietal regions.

Roberts (1966, p. 22) explains anatomical, physiological, and psychological considerations in speech in this way. Comprehension of speech takes place when auditory impulses are transmitted to the auditory cortex of both hemispheres and subsequently transmitted to interact with activity in the central speech system; Broca's, the supplementary motor, and temporoparietal regions (the most important area) and interrelated subcortical structures (probably the pulvinar of the thalamus and other areas) make up the speech system. Also considered important, with respect to the system's focusing upon auditory stimuli, is the participation of the ascending reticular activating system. Comprehension of written words, on the other hand, takes place when visual impulses are transmitted to the visual cortex of both hemispheres and subsequently transmitted to interact with the central speech system (interaction with the auditory system is also probable).

Production of speech or writing (both viewed simply as different forms of verbal behavior) takes place when neurorrheuma (mechanism of the energy source is still unknown) causes impulses from the speech center system to interact with those of the motor system.

Hemispheral Differences and the Limbic System

Additional information relating to the neuro-phylo-ontogenesis of the speech system has been offered by Geschwind (Roberts, 1966, pp. 26–30). Geschwind referred to work being done on the question of anatomical differences in the two hemispheres. In short, findings tend to indicate that there are differences in Heschl's gyri (cortical structures involved in hearing) in the temporal lobes of both hemispheres. This is in contrast to the bilateral similarity of Heschl's gyri in monkeys, which incidentally appear in pattern to be like those usually found in the right hemisphere of man. According to Geschwind, if these differences do, in fact, exist, the probable reason is that Wernicke's area has grown to the point where it has pushed the auditory cortex forward. Geschwind also indicated that the posterior inferior parietal region is more developed in man than in any other animal.

Geschwind, in discussing the anatomical background of learning in the monkey, makes interesting references to the limbic * system, inter-modal or cross-modal associations (associations between stimuli in two different sensory modalities), and the development of language in man.

In teaching a monkey to select a certain visual form, the monkey receives a piece of food only if he selects the form desired by the experimenter. When successful, the monkey has formed an association between a visual stimulus and a food stimulus, or monkey-learning in this instance is the result of a visual-limbic association. Such a task is usually easy for a monkey and, in fact, the monkey's brain appears anatomically designed for such activity (largest number of connections of the visual system are with the limbic system). Monkeys also form tactile-limbic associations and auditory-limbic associations, that is, as-sociations between other non-limbic and limbic modalities. It appears that what is difficult for the monkey is to form an association between two non-limbic stimuli.

Such non-limbic associations are relatively easy for man and this is usually attributed to the fact that man utilizes "verbal mediation." Geschwind indicated that this means that man ". . . learns in the visual experiment to choose the object named 'circle'; when the tactile experiment is done he again chooses the object named 'circle.'" Gesch-wind (Roberts, 1966, p. 30) believes, however, that, "What is impor-tant is not that we need language in order to have cross-modal associations: it is rather that in order to develop language we must be able to form non-limbic cross-modal associations." Hence, man learns to name objects by associating the sight or feel of it with a particular auditory stimulus (its name); however, it is just this kind of non-limbic, cross-modal association which is a problem for the monkey to make.

It is expected that as the child begins to form non-limbic, cross-modal associations, he begins to show language acquisition, which may be viewed as a special kind of non-limbic, cross-modal association. Geschwind believes that the basis for forming non-limbic, intermodal associations is related to the development in man of the angular gyrus region. He feels that since the angular gyrus region is situated at the junction of the visual, auditory, and somesthetic association regions, it is well-suited to function as an association area of association areas. Hence, the angular gyrus region may be viewed as the anatomical substrate for man's ability to make non-limbic, cross-modal transfers.

---

* ". . . that portion of the brain which connects with the regions in which are represented both the subjective and objective manifestations of behavior related to the survival of the individual or the species—the motor aspects of rage, flight and sexual behavior, the feelings of hunger or thirst with the corresponding feelings of satiation, and other similar behaviors and emotions."

CEREBRAL MATURATION

A discussion of the neuro-ontogenesis of the speech system would be incomplete without a discussion of the connection between cerebral maturation and oral language development. In this regard, much in the way of recent and most interesting material has been published by Lenneberg (1966a, 1966b, 1967).

Lenneberg (1966b) in a recent chapter asks the question why children regularly begin to speak between 18 and 28 months of life. After commenting on the contributions of "training," "need," and "pleasure," Lenneberg (1966b, p. 219) states, ". . . the most important differences between the prelanguage and postlanguage phases of development originate in the growing individual and not in the external world or in changes in the availability of stimuli."

Lenneberg bases his discussion of whether the onset of language may be best attributed to a maturational process by referring to four criteria of "maturationally controlled emergence of behavior." In short, Lenneberg (1966b, p. 235) describes these criteria as: "regularity in onset, differential use of environmental stimulation with growth, independence from use, and superfluousness of practice."

Below are some of the reasons Lenneberg (1966b, pp. 221–235) offers to support his belief that language-learning is apparently a consequence of maturation (assuming the existence of an adequate environment). (1) The normally interlinking sequential development of oral language and the development of functions more easily connected to physical maturation such as gait and motor coordination. (2) The finding that the interrelationships between language development and other developments is frequently maintained even when the whole maturational process is slowed because of various types of mental retardation. (3) The regularity in the emergence of language (e.g., according to Lenneberg, approximately 100 per cent of children acquire single words by 22 months; and two-word phrases by 36 months). (4) The uncovering of no evidence that intensive language stimulation can accelerate language development in a child who is maturationally still a toddling infant.

Lenneberg (1966b, p. 235) indicates, ". . . Complementary to the question of how old a child must be before he can use the environment for language acquisition is that of how young he must be before it is too late to acquire speech and language." Of course, information with reference to age limitation on language acquisition as well as to onset of language acquisition should be of special interest to speech specialists concerned with the cerebral palsied.

Lenneberg offers the following evidence that primary acquisition of language depends on a developmental phase which is outgrown at about puberty (2 to about 13 years). (1) At about the time cerebral lateralization becomes well established (about puberty), symptoms of acquired aphasia tend to become irreversible. (2) In a group of retardates (Down's Syndrome), language-learning ceases after puberty. (3) Profoundly deaf children have a much better chance of good speech if amplication and training begin as close to the age of two as possible.

More specifically related to a discussion of cerebral maturation are Lenneberg's findings on the physical states of the brain before, during, and after the period of primary language acquisition. Lenneberg (1967, pp. 158–170) has collected anatomical, histological, biochemical, and electrophysiological data on the maturation of the brain. In short, it was shown that in all those aspects of brain maturation studied, about 60 per cent of the mature values are reached before the onset of speech (about two years of age), then the maturation rate slows down and the brain reaches its mature state by the close of the period of primary language acquisition.

EVOLUTION OF ORAL COMMUNICATION

Following is an attempt to outline the phylogenesis of human oral communication. It should be noted that the author will describe this "development" with a view toward how the concepts selected may contribute to the next chapter's discussion of neurospeech therapy.

As to knowledge concerning the origin of speech in man, Hoijer (1966, p. 232) recently stated that there is ". . . no evidence in the form of·archeological remains of early stages of language evolution, though we must assume that language, like other aspects of culture underwent a period of evolutionary development." In the same vein, Simon (1957, pp. 8–23), in a scholarly discussion of the development of speech in the race, stated that ". . . Speech, practically alone of all man's activities, has left no record of its origin and development." (Simon, 1957, p. 8)

Following are instructive points made by Simon in his discussion. (1) Information on the beginnings of speech in man must be inferred from the structure of primitive men and from the records of the kinds of life they lived. (2) Primitive man probably gestured and used calls and yells much before he began to use speech sounds. "The transition from the merely representative use of preverbal sounds to the arbitrary symbols of speech may well have been most gradual." (Simon, 1957, p. 10) (3) About 30 to 40 million years ago, one division of primate vertebrates (the one that did not remain in the trees to evolve into monkeys and apes) slowly developed terrestrial living patterns and evolved into man. Over the next millions of years of increased terrestrial living came the bipedal posture and the development of manual dexterity and hence freedom of the mouth from grasping and manipulative activities. This type of bipedal-manual development also meant corresponding changes in the sensorimotor areas of the cortex. Freedom of the mouth allowed oral and throat structures to slowly evolve into the various organs needed to support the speech process. The brain also underwent a progressive increase in size and complexity. (4) The archeological remains of "Java man" and "Peking man," thought to be contemporaneous about a million years ago, indicate ". . . usuable speech structures and probably just adequate brains . . ." to justify the inference that these primitive men used a human type of oral communication. (5) Some improvement in speech equipment was shown by "Heidelberg man" (approximately 500,000 years ago); greatly improved equipment for speech was shown by "Neanderthal man" (100,000 to 150,000 years ago); and "Cro-Magnon man" (about 50,000 years ago), who was similar to modern man in appearance, showed through his cultural remains ". . . considerable use of his fully developed speech mechanism."

Distance between man was no doubt another factor behind the need for and development of oral communication. As population and group living expanded, increasingly more individuals were present in man's living space or biosphere and something that might be called the "communisphere" developed. The concept of "communisphere" relates to the rise in the need to communicate when men are within about 12 feet of each other. Distances of an arm's length, more or less, invite person-to-person communication, while distances somewhat beyond are more conducive to person-to-group communication.

The points of particular interest in this phyletic tracing of speech, with respect to the central purpose of Part Two of this book, are: man's assumption of the bipedal posture; man's development of manual dexterity; the freeing of man's mouth from crude grasping and manipulative activities; the associated changes in man's sensory and motor areas of the cortex; and the development of the communisphere. It is obvious that many of the developments which appear pertinent to the phylogenesis of speech are recapitulated in the ontogenesis of speech.

Theories on the Origin of Oral Language

In order to theorize about the beginnings of oral communication, it is of course necessary to base a great deal of the discussion on various inferences and extrapolations. As might be expected, throughout the history of man many kinds of explanations have been offered for how speech began. The author will briefly describe speech theories here which, for the greater part, actually represent categories of theories.

The term *"natural theories"* could be used to describe all those theories which posit that some type of natural and inherent relationship exists between oral symbols and the things, acts, and so on, which they represent.

"Onomatopoetic theories" are all those theories which view the source of many words as oral imitations of the sounds made by the things they represent.

"Vocal emotion theories" are those which indicate that the source of words are the reflexive utterances made during various kinds of emotional experiences.

"Common effort theories" are those which indicate that words emerged from the vocalizations made by men engaged in group physical effort in order to synchronize their physical efforts.

"Social pressure and control theories" are those which indicate that as man joined groups for purposes of safety and economy of effort, and also desired group control, and so forth, the need for various types of oral signals and symbols grew.

"Body language theories" are those which view words as oral gestures growing out of bodily gestures.

"Vocal play theories" would represent all those theories which suggest that certain involuntary utterances or play vocalizations became associated with various acts.

"Cortical emergence theories" are those which state that oral symbols are the product of the development of the cerebrum which, in turn, is responsible for the meaningful linking and associating of neuromotor patterns responsible for already present reflexive sounds.

The *"multiple sources or combination theories"* are those which indicate more than one source for the origin of word-noises. Hence, a combination theory such as the *body language-onomatopoetic-vocal emotion theory* might be offered to explain the sources of different groups of words. This multiple-source orientation appears most interesting and could be viewed as receiving support from Van Riper's discussion of the different functions of speech (1963, pp. 2–11).

Functions of speech, as viewed by Van Riper, include the role of speech in the formulation of thought, in communication, in emotional expression, in social control, and in the identification of self. In short, the role of speech in the formulation of thought implies that a good deal of thinking by those of us who possess speech consists of covert speech behavior, or inner speech; the role of speech as communication describes the utility of speech in the transmission of information, that is, in the sending and receiving of messages; the role of speech as social control means the use of speech as a way to manipulate others or to help control the environment; the role of speech as emotional expression means the use of speech as a way of letting others know how the speaker is feeling about himself or others; and the role of speech as self-expression means the use of speech as a way of identifying and exhibiting the self or calling attention to the self.

It is proposed, then, that if in fact speech has different functions, it may be assumed that the numerous types of word-noises of which it is composed might also have different sources.

Multi-source, Progressive Differentiation and Selection Theory of Speech

On the basis of the preceding information, and on the basis of information available on the ontogenesis of oral language, the author will present an outline of the stages in the phylogenesis of oral language. The description, in simple terms, will be based on the assumption that there were multiple sources for meaningful human vocalizations; that speech behavior, like other sensory-motor behaviors, proceeded from more generalized, relatively undifferentiated behaviors to more specific highly differentiated behaviors; and, finally, that selection took place of those speech behaviors which were most efficient. Each stage of the phylogenesis of oral language will include a discussion of pertinent bodily activity and associated vocal behavior.

Pre-language. It is believed that when early, pre-language man was moved in some way, for example, social pressure, emotion, or the need for action, he used relatively unorganized bodily, hands, head, face, and mouth movements in association with unorganized vocalizations; that is, he used generalized, undifferentiated bodily and vocal responses.

Body-Head Language. Gradually, in the presence of changes in bodily structures and with appropriate stimuli, there was a first step toward progressive differentiation and selection of communication behavior. Hands, face, mouth and vocalization behavior remained relatively unorganized, but more general bodily and head movements became expressive. So that, for example, man used certain posturings and growls and screams (primitive phonatory and articulatory behavior) to indicate his impending attack behavior, analogous to the attack or preparatory "spring" postures and growls of numerous present-day predatory animals.

Hands-Face Language. Next, this body-head, unorganized vocalization stage underwent further differentiation and early man began to produce meaningful bilateral hand movements and facial expressions in association with more organized vocalization (vocalizations whose acoustic dimensions were associated with pain, pleasure, or anger). At this time, hands-face language became "figure" and body-head language became "ground."

Face-Hand Language. With the further passage of time, man developed finer unilateral hand gestures, increased his repertoire of facial expressions, and began to vary not only his phonatory patterns but also his articulatory patterns, so that articulatory patterns used to imitate animal sounds or other sounds in the environment began to be manifested. In short, there was a transition from emphasis on a crude hand communication to an emphasis on finer hand communication and an increase in facial and articulatory activity.

Mouth Language. Finally, in modern man we may observe not only appropriate and complex unilateral hand movements and facial expressions and controlled phonatory patterns but the use of an arbitrary acoustical-temporal code or the symbolic use of vocal sounds. At this present stage of development then, mouth language has become "figure" and body-head, hands-face, and face-hand systems of communication have become "ground."

Before concluding this section of the chapter, it should be interesting to comment on some of the phyletic reflections in present-day man's speech development and speech behavior. For example, many stages in oral language ontogenesis are suggestive of many of the hypotheses advanced for stages in oral language phylogenesis. These include: (1) the relation between the development of the bipedal stage and the beginnings of true words; and (2) the progressive differentiation of bodily activities, hands and face activities, and vocalization.

Further, certain bodily, hand, facial, and vocalization behaviors used during different oral communication situations may be viewed as "vestigial" forms of oral language which were more appropriate and more dominant during other times in man's speech history. For example, during moments of heated argument, present-day man may be noted to accompany his speaking with gross body movements, he may make excessive and irregular hand movements, he may make grosser than usual facial expressions, lose control over the pitch, quality, loudness and time dimensions of his voice (i.e., he may scream or shout), and his articulation may suffer as well as his choice of words.

Numerous other communicative situations elicit reflexive and reactive sounds as well as stimulus sounds of which many may be viewed as vestigial communicative behaviors. The most obvious of these possible vestigial sound forms are those that may be termed signal reactions. These would include screams and cries of infants, children, and adults heard during sorrow, terror, and life-threatening situations. Other categories of vestigial-like sounds include: the "a-ha" group which may be uttered during moments of insight or discovery; the "h-rr" group which may be uttered during moments of anger or hostility; the "mm" group which may be uttered during pleasant moments or moments of contentment; the "ow" group which may be uttered during moments of pain; the "ee" group which may be uttered during moments of general excitement, and so forth.

In summary, one of the important purposes of Chapter Four is to prepare the reader for concepts to be found in the last chapter of the book relating to speech system arrestment, retardation, or dissolution in cerebral palsy and treatment for such involvement. A recapitulation of major points made in Chapter Four follows:

1. The development of propositional speech and the development of bipedal head, neck, and trunk balance appear to be approximately concurrent phenomena in the normal child.

2. Oroneuromotor maturation, as described by the emergence and extinction of certain reflexes and reactions categorized under the headings of protective, vegetative, and emotional reflexes, and its possible significance to articulatory behavior and articulatory disorders is a necessary area of study by speech pathologists.

3. Important to speech functioning in man is the development of the "uncommitted cortex" in the left hemisphere, the development of the angular gyrus region, and the ability of man to make non-limbic, cross-modal associations.

4. It is estimated that early man began to make some form of meaningful speech about one million years ago. The evolution of speech in man appears related to the development of the bipedal posture, manual dexterity, the liberation of the mouth from use in crude grasping and manipulative activities, and the development of the communisphere.

5. Categories of theories on the beginnings of speech in man include natural theories, onomatopoetic theories, social pressure and control theories, common effort theories, body language theories, vocal play theories, cortical emergence theories, and multiple-sources theories.

6. A multi-source, progressive differentiation and selection theory of the phylogenesis of speech is presented and includes the following stages: pre-language, body-head language, hands-face language, face-hand language and, finally, mouth language.

REFERENCES

André-Thomas, Chesni, Y. and Dargassies, S., Saint-Anne *The Neurological Examination of the Infant.* London: National Spastics Society, 1960.

Brain, R. W. *Diseases of the Nervous System.* London: Oxford University Press, 1955.

Hoijer, H. "The problem of Primitive Languages" in Edward C. Carterette (Ed.), *Brain Function: Speech, Language, and Communication.* Berkeley and Los Angeles: University of California Press, 1966.

Hooker, D. *The Prenatal Origin of Behavior.* Lawrence, Kansas: University of Kansas Press, 1952.

Illingworth, R. S. *An Introduction to Developmental Assessment in the First Year.* London: National Spastics Society, 1962.

Lenneberg, E. H. *Biological Foundations of Language.* New York: John Wiley and Sons, Inc., 1967.

Lenneberg, E. H. "Speech Development: Its Anatomical and Physiological Concomitants" in Edward C. Carterette (Ed.), *Brain Function: Speech, Language, and Communication.* Berkeley and Los Angeles: University of California Press, 1966a.

Lenneberg, E. H. "The Natural History of Language" in Frank Smith and George A. Miller (Eds.), *The Genesis of Language.* Cambridge: The M.I.T. Press, 1966b.

Meader, Mary H. "The effect of disturbances in the developmental processes upon emergent specificity of function." *J. Speech Dis.,* 5, 1940, 211–219.

Miller, F. R. and Sherrington, C. S. "Some observations on the buccopharyngeal stage of reflex deglutition." *Quart J. Exp. Physiol.,* 9, 1915, 147–186.

Mysak, E. D. "Significance of neurophysiological orientation to cerebral palsy habilitation." *J. Speech Hearing Dis.,* 24, 1959, 221–230.

Mysak, E. D. "Dysarthria and oropharyngeal reflexology: a review." *J. Speech Hearing Dis.,* 28, 1963, 252–260.

Mysak, E. D. "Reflex Therapy and Cerebral Palsy Habilitation" in William T. Daley (Ed.), *Speech and Language Therapy with the Cerebral Palsied Child.* Washington, D.C.: The Catholic University of America Press, 1965.

Peiper, A. *Cerebral Function in Infancy and Childhood,* New York: Consultants Bureau, 1963.

Penfield, W. *Speech, Perception and the Uncommitted Cortex* in John C. Eccles (Ed.), *Brain and Conscious Experience.* New York: Springer-Verlag, 1966.

Penfield, W. and Roberts, L. *Speech and Brain Mechanisms.* Princeton: Princeton University Press, 1959.

Prechtl, H. F. R. "The directed head-turning response and allied movements of the human baby." *Behavior,* 13, 1958, 212–242.

Roberts, L. "Central Brain Mechanisms in Speech" in Edward C. Carterette (Ed.), *Brain Function: Speech, Language, and Communication.* Berkeley and Los Angeles: University of California Press, 1966.

Schwartz, A. B. "Congenital laryngeal stridor-speculations regarding its origin." *Pediatrics,* 27, 477–479, 1961.

Simon, C. T. "The Development of Speech" in Lee Edward Travis (Ed.), *Handbook of Speech Pathology.* New York: Appleton-Century-Crofts, Inc., 1957.

Thomson, J. "On the lip-reflex (mouth phenomenon) of newborn children." *Rev. Neurol. Psychiat.,* 1, 1903, 145–148.

Travis, L. E. *Speech Pathology.* New York: D. Appleton-Century Co., 1931.

Van Riper, C. *Speech Correction.* Englewood Cliffs: Prentice-Hall, Inc., 1963.

CHAPTER FIVE

Neurospeech Therapy

The last chapter of the book will identify, from a neuroevolutional standpoint, the respiratory-phonatory-articulatory complex of the cerebral palsied and will also present the principles of a speech habilitation program.

RESPIRATORY-PHONATORY-ARTICULATORY DISORDER IN CEREBRAL PALSY

It may be recalled that in Chapter One the major symptoms of cerebral palsy were defined as reflections of disturbed neuro-ontogenesis. In terms of Jacksonian concepts, at least two groups of symptoms were identified—that is, negative and positive symptoms. The negative symptoms were viewed as loss or defect of function symptoms related to involvement of the least organized, most complex, and least automatic centers of the central nervous system, while the positive, or involuntary activity symptoms, were viewed as related to involvement or release of the more organized, less complex, and more automatic centers of the central nervous system.

It is proposed that the frequently exhibited respiratory-phonatory-articulatory complex in cerebral palsy may also be viewed from the standpoint of nervous system arrestment, retardation, or dissolution, and duplex symptomatology.

Neuroevolutional Interpretation of Speech System Problems

Respiratory involvement in congenital or acquired cerebral palsy may include: paretic thoracic and abdominal muscles; shallow inspiratory-expiratory cycles causing a reduced air supply; an increased number and range of breaths per minute (bpm); a conflict between inspiratory and expiratory phases, or so-called "oppositional" breathing; predominantly abdominal breathing patterns; and the use of predominantly vegetative breathing patterns for both vegetative and speech purposes.

With reference to respiratory activity, paretic respiratory musculature may be viewed basically as negative symptomatology, while an increased bpm, predominant abdominal breathing activity and the use of vegetative for speech breathing patterns, may be viewed as reflections of positive symptoms.

Phonatory involvement in the cerebral palsied may include decreased ability to abduct and adduct the folds, involuntary open-close activity, and periodic over-close behavior.

Abductor-adductor dysfunctioning could be viewed primarily as part of the negative symptomatology, while involuntary open-close and over-close activity could be viewed primarily as positive symptomatology. The over-close tendency, in particular, might represent the irregular retention or release of the primitive glottic-closing reflex described in Chapter Four.

Articulatory deficits in the cerebral palsied may include reduced ability to effect movements of the lips, mandible, tongue, and of the velopharyngeal area, involuntary movements of these organs, and the manifestation of motor patterns suggestive of infantile lip, mouth-opening, biting, and suckling reflexes.

As with the two previous categories, reduced motility of the articulators would be interpreted as part of the paralytic or negative symptomatology, while the involuntary movements, and the more specific retention or release of various infantile feeding reflexes, would be interpreted as positive symptoms.

Review of Pertinent Literature

In the ensuing portion of the chapter, certain information from the literature will be offered in support of the concept that retention or release phenomena are often important accompaniments to cerebral palsy speech problems. For purposes of simplicity, "neurogenic articulatory disorders" will refer to those cases of dysarthria where there are negative and(or) positive neurologic symptoms. "Reflexogenic articulatory disturbances" will refer to speech deficits associated with nonparalytic cases where only retention or release phenomena may be observable. It should be understood that the positive oral symptoms found in certain speech cases may be incomplete or residual rather than full responses.

Neurogenic Articulatory Disorders. The writer has observed the presence of the complicating persistence of infantile reflexes in cases of dysarthria associated with cerebral palsy. Cephalic, rooting, mouth-opening, lip, biting, chewing, suckling, smiling, and laughter reflexes in various combinations and of varying strengths have all been detected. As a specific example of dysarthria with negative and positive features, the negative aspect may be represented by the child's inability to move the articulators into position for the [f] in "farm," while the positive aspect may be represented by mandibular over-extension (elicitation of mouth-opening reflex) during the attempt to produce the [a] in "farm." In addition, Clement and Twitchell (1959) have discussed the avoiding response and the grasp reflex in cerebral palsy; their descriptions of the manifestations of these responses in the speech mechanisms of athetotic and spastic children are suggestive of retained rooting and lip reflexes. Such phenomena may also be observed as part of the dysarthria of many of the degenerative and traumatic CNS involvements. Support for this may be found in Brain's statement that the "sucking reflex is lost after infancy but may reappear in states of severe cerebral degeneration, for example, the presenile and senile dementias" (1955, pp. 42–43).

In response to the author's observations on positive symptoms in dysarthria associated with cerebral palsy, Sheppard (1964) studied 51 cerebral palsied children for the incidence of infantile cranio-oropharyngeal motor patterns and their relationship to age, feeding competence, speech intelligibility, and progress in speech therapy. She found that infantile patterns were frequently found in the subjects and that an inverse relationship existed between the number of patterns elicited in an individual and speech and feeding proficiency, progress in speech therapy, and age. Witkop and Henry (1963) in a study of children with Sjogren-Larsson syndrome also found not only speech and language problems but also the persistence of vigorous sucking and rooting reflexes at age five.

In the area of adult neurologic disorder and dysarthria, Grewel (1957) reported the tendency for speech behavior in one of his patients to be accompanied by yawning, biting, and snout movements of the lips and mouth. Personal clinical observation confirms the occasional appearance of oral release phenomena in patients with parkinsonism, CVA, and other adult neurologic disorders. Further, Schneider (1938) has reported different degrees and combinations of echolalia, echopraxia, forced prehension reflex, and suction reflex in cases with vascular, toxic, infectious, and psychotic backgrounds.

To cite a specific language example of negative and positive manifestations, Jackson, in explaining the meaningless recurring jargon, swearing, words and phrases uttered by certain aphasics, stated,

> To say that the disease "caused" these utterances—a positive condition—is absurd, for the disease is destruction of nervous arrangements, and that could not cause a man to do something; it has enough

to answer for in leaving him unable to speak . . . it is an error to ascribe such positive symptoms as the recurring utterances in speechless men, the erroneous words uttered by those who have defect of speech . . . to negative lesions, to loss or to defect of function. These positive mental symptoms arise during activity of lower centres or lower nervous arrangements which have escaped injury . . . (Head, 1915, pp. 154–155).

Reflexogenic Articulatory Disorders. As evidence for the presence of infantile oral phenomena in cases where no apparent neuropathology exists, there may be observed the re-emergence of lip and suckling reflexes in normal older children during drowsy states when higher brain mechanisms diminish in activity. Related to this phenomenon is the presumed origin of some of the involuntary movements noticed in the oral musculature of inebriated individuals; accordingly, portions of the "dysarthria" of intoxication may possibly be attributed to transient release phenomena.

Oral tics suggestive of lip and rooting reflexes are sometimes seen in emotionally disturbed individuals and, if present, may add to the speech symptoms of some of these individuals. In this regard, Coriat (1943) has described the act of stuttering as an extension into adult life of infantile nursing behavior. Mouth phenomena suggestive of release symptoms are often discernible in some nonparalytic aged individuals and may possibly contribute to their articulatory deterioration. Lip pursing and retracting in the manner of a lip reflex is seen as many elders prepare to utter or when they are between utterances; this is especially apparent if they are edentulous.

Finally, it has been observed and reported that suckling reflexes have been elicited in some children and adults with interdental lisps. It would appear that their protruding tongue activity during speech may be related to their retention of suckling-like oral behavior. In this connection, "visceral swallowing" has recently received considerable attention in the literature, and many of its forms might be described as representing infantile suckle-swallow activity. Many possible speech sound substitutions have also been reported (Ward, *et al.*, 1961) to be associated with such a swallow pattern.

Granted that some of the observations described here need further clarification, it is nevertheless felt that oral retention and release phenomena are present in certain individuals with nonparalytic articulatory problems, and that these phenomena, directly or indirectly, may serve to hamper their articulatory efforts.

This review indicates that clinicians who evaluate paralytic articulatory problems should consider not only the particular articulatory muscle deficits and concomitant phonetic lapses, but should also assess the degree to which positive symptom phenomena might be involved. Difficulty in swallowing, accompanied by drooling, and disturbances of the palatal and pharyngeal reflexes with accompanying nasality should also be noted; the connections between these observations should be obvious.

Similarly, when confronted with misarticulations of unknown origin, it is advisable to check routinely for the possible persistence of infantile oral reflexes. Many cases of interdental lisp, rhotacism, lambdacism, dentalization of lingua-alveolar sounds, labiodental deviations, labiodental production of bilabials, and excessive lingual protrusion of linguadental sounds may be found to possess contributory infantile oral phenomena.

With regard to the last statement, the author has periodically identified residual rooting or jaw deviating patterns in children with lateralized sibilants, and lip phenomena with reduced differentiation between the tongue and lip in cases of bilabialized rhotacism and lambdacism.

BASES OF A NEUROSPEECH THERAPY APPROACH

The bases of a neurospeech therapy approach to the speech disorder in cerebral palsy are drawn from the following neuro-phylo-onto-genetic concepts:

1. The evolution of speech in man is related to the development of the bipedal posture, manual dexterity, the liberation of the mouth from use in crude grasping and manipulative activities, and the development of the communisphere. The ontogenetic reflection of this phyletic heritage is observed when noting the relationship of these phenomena with the beginning of true speech in the infant. True speech in the human is approximately concurrent with the development of bipedal head, neck, and trunk balance, the use of a preferred hand, the extinction of infantile feeding reflexes, and the need to communicate.

2. Sensorimotor behavior in the developing human proceeds from generalized, un-coordinated responses towards increased specificity, differentiation, and selectivity in behavior, all as a function of age. Related developmental concepts include: (a) the simpler the function the more rapid its development; (b) the more complex the function, usually the slower it is to develop; (c) the coordination of large muscles precedes the coordination of small muscles; and (d) the life of an organism is marked with periods when it will profit most from certain kinds of environmental stimulation.

3. Phylo-ontogenesis of speech in man has many stages. It is proposed that at least a body-head stage, a hands-face stage, a face-hand stage and, finally, a mouth stage may be identified.

PRINCIPLES OF NEUROSPEECH THERAPY

Neurospeech therapy for the speech disorder in cerebral palsy is designed to help the child to control and regulate the nervous energy required for the proper innervation of his speech system. It should be noted that this section of the chapter will be concerned with describing primarily the principles of the approach and will not attempt to provide specific techniques for the many individual problems that children with cerebral palsy may exhibit. Knowledge of general principles and strategies should enable the clinician to develop the techniques needed to suit the various individual cases.

Goals in neurospeech therapy should, of course, be planned only after careful consideration of the particular child's level of neurodevelopment. Contrary to this concept, goals in conventional speech therapy programs are often set in accordance with the chronological age or mental age rather than in accordance with these factors as well as neurophysiological considerations. Further, the procedures and techniques described below are designed to ameliorate the quality or the respiratory-phonatory-articulatory involvement; the clinician should also give appropriate attention, wherever indicated, to the quantity or oral language involvement. With respect to oral language development, the clinician should be concerned with whether there is a relatively intact left cerebral hemisphere or, at least, one intact hemisphere. He should also be interested in any information concerning the cortico-thalamic tracts of the speech system and the angular gyri. Prognosis for oral language development should, in general, be poorer in cases of bilateral hemispheric involvement and involvement of the angular gyri and cortico-thalamic tracts of the speech system. Finally, in planning programs to facilitate oral language acquisition, attention should be given to factors such as stimulating intermodal, non-limbic associations and sensory modality hierarchy and sensory synthesis; and to the understanding that primary language acquisition is thought to take place between two and 13 years of age. For a sample form which may be used in evaluating the speech system, the reader should refer to Appendix B.

The general goal in neurospeech therapy, which is an organismic rather than a speech organ approach, is to stimulate the highest level of speech system neuro-ontogenesis by (1) restraining positive symptoms such as infantile breathing and laryngeal activity and infantile oropharyngeal vegetative and emotional reflexes, and (2) facilitating speech system sensorimotor integration at the highest CNS centers.

Positive Symptom Inhibiting Postures

The speech clinician must first analyze his client's general system to determine those particular supine, side-lying, and sitting positions which tend to normalize muscle tone in the respiratory-phonatory-articulatory system. As indicated previously, these techniques usually involve aligning the head, neck, arms, thorax, and legs in ways which are contrary to infantile positions, resisting the build-up of muscle tone upon the accomplishment of such positioning, recognizing the subsequent "normalizing" of muscle tone, and performing all aspects of neurospeech therapy during these periods. Such periods of more normal muscle tone vary in length but should be found to gradually increase with time.

Such restraining postures should allow for more normal tactile-proprioceptive feedbacks as well as for a higher-center integration of these feedbacks. Depending on the particular child's level of neuromaturation (e.g., supine, sitting), two or three postures conducive to more normal respiration and voicing should be acquired by the child.

Bipedal Head and Neck and Thoracic Balance

Since true words are usually uttered at about the time the child's CNS allows for a bipedal form of head and neck and thoracic balance, it would be well if the clinician worked toward establishing this form of balance with the cerebral palsied child.

Here the clinician should attempt to restrain infantile reflexes such as the symmetrical and asymmetrical tonic neck reflexes and the tonic labyrinthine reflexes, and to elicit reflexes such as the protective-extensor-thrust of the arms reaction, the precipitation reflex, the labyrinthine righting reflex acting on the head, and the body righting reflex acting on the body. Equilibrium reactions in supine and prone, in side-lying, in two-point, three-point, and four-point crawling positions, and in the sitting position should also be stimulated and established.

Hemispheral Dominance

The connection between a dominant hemisphere and speech functioning appears rather well established. Neurotherapy techniques which may contribute to the establishment of a speech dominant hemisphere include: (1) in general, stimulation which facilitates over-all neuromaturation, for example, development from brain stem to midbrain and above levels should contribute to the development of a speech dominant hemisphere; (2) elicitation of righting and equilibrium reactions with emphasis on right-sided reactions, for example: when eliciting the neck righting reflex and the body righting reflex acting on the body, the majority of the movements should be toward the right side; when eliciting equilibrium reactions in side-lying, sitting, and standing, the child's left hand should be used more frequently as the "pull-hand" while the right limbs are left free to respond to the shifting center of gravity of the body; (3) facilitation of standing or reaching with the use of the left foot and hand as stabilizing and(or) "push-off" limbs; and (4) the encouragement of the use of the right foot and hand as lead limbs in, for example, stepping or reaching out.

The mother, occupational therapist, and teacher also assist in establishing laterality and, hopefully, may help contribute to the development of a speech dominant hemisphere.

Speech System Differentiation

Following developmental sequences, the clinician facilitates the progressive differentiation of the respiratory-phonatory-articulatory system. Toward this end, he attempts to differentiate the thorax and head from the rest of the body, or the upper-half from the lower-half of the body, the head and neck from the thorax, the articulators from the head and neck, and, finally, the articulators from each other. Differentiation techniques are employed by first positioning the individual appropriately, and then, for example, passively moving the upper body by bending it forward and backward, from side to side, and through a rotatory movement, while stablizing the lower half of the body. These procedures are followed until the individual is able to effect upper body movement independent of lower body movement, first with assistance, and finally unassisted.

The head and neck are similarly differentiated from the thorax by first passively moving the head and neck laterally (rotating the head around the long axis so that the chin is positioned over the shoulder), ventroflexing and dorsiflexing it, and bending the head in an ear-to-shoulder fashion. Again, these maneuvers are imposed until the child is able to perform them with and without assistance.

Next, the clinician works toward differentiating the articulators from the head. The goal here is to get the child to the point where he can spread and pucker the lips, where he can flex and extend the mandible, and where he can protrude and retrude the tongue—each movement being independent of associated head and neck movements. Finally, the articulators are differentiated from each other. For example, the mandible may be flexed and extended passively while preventing associated movements of the lips and tongue (hands as well as tongue depressors may be needed to prevent the tendency for associated articulator movements of the articulators) and until the child is able to effect voluntarily rather independent and isolated mandibular movements. Similar procedures are used to facilitate differentiated lip and tongue movements.

Speech system differentiation has been achieved when the child is able to move the head and neck and the various articulators independent of the rest of the body and of each other. Of course, depending on the individual child, varying degrees of such speech system differentiation will be possible. Progress in this goal should be found to contribute to improved phonatory and articulatory behavior.

Oral Reflex Inhibition and Facilitation

In line with neuroevolutional concepts, oral reflex inhibition and facilitation procedures are designed to stimulate oroneuromotor maturation from the point where the oral mechanism is used for crude grasping and manipulative activities, such as during holding and biting nipples and teething rings and during vegetative functioning, to the point where the mechanism is able to produce highly differentiated and selective speech articulatory events.

Oropharyngeal Reflex Facilitation. In cases of congenital problems where essential feeding reflexes are weak or absent—for example, rooting, lip, mouth-opening, biting, suckling, chewing, and swallowing reflexes—these should be stimulated. As previously indicated, it is believed that such reflexes may serve as background activity for the emerging movements which are necessary for complex articulatory behavior. Excitation of the various feeding reflexes is done by applying the appropriate stimulus and then initiating and guiding the expected response. In this way, it is hoped that the particular chain synaptic pathway necessary for the motor activity being sought may be established and developed. In accordance with the natural sequence, these infantile reflexes, after being stimulated and after serving their vegetative functions, should eventually be restrained and replaced by higher forms of oroneuromotor activity.

Designed for both congenital and acquired dysarthrias are procedures for counteracting drooling, the often encountered "jaw-droop" (both of which may be hampering articulation), and hypernasality.

In instances of drooling associated with dysphagia, attempts at exciting a more normal rate of swallowing (about two swallows per minute) may be made by: (1) stimulating the back of the tongue or palate with a small tongue depressor; (2) directing a stream of water from an eye dropper against the posterior pharyngeal wall while the head is in moderate dorsiflexion; and (3) encouraging gentle token coughing. These procedures may be carried out by providing one or two of the adequate stimuli every 30 seconds for short periods of time two or three times a day. Efforts at relieving hypernasality, due to incompetency of the velopharyngeal closure mechanism associated with disturbed palatal and pharyngeal reflexes, may be made by regular, periodic attempts at stimulating the palatal, pharyngeal (especially mesial movement of the lateral pharyngeal musculature) and yawning reflexes. Velar stroking accompanying these efforts may be found helpful. Finally, the "jaw-droop" condition may be helped by making use of the mandibular or jaw-jerk reflex. It is elicited by tapping the chin of the lowered jaw. A brief reflexive elevation of the jaw characterizes the response pattern.

Oropharyngeal Reflex Inhibition. Since involuntary movements of the head and articulators in response to chest, neck, jaw, and cheek stimulation are often seen in children with cerebral palsy, and since these may be triggered inadvertently causing further interference with articulatory efforts, attempts at restraining these responses should be made. Similarly, since the frequently overactive smiling and laughter reflexes often complicate athetotic dysarthria, these reflexes should also be desensitized. Tolerance to stimulation and eventual adaptation may be gradually attained by regular, periodic handling and later self-handling of sensitive thoracic and head and neck areas, as well as by stimulating affected areas and resisting the accompanying involuntary movement. Relative to the laughing reflex, planned periodic excitation of sustained laughing responses may be noticed to diminish the intensity of the reflex over a period of time.

Lastly, persisting or retained cephalic, rooting, lip, mouth-opening, biting, and suckling reactions which are considered to be compounding an articulatory problem should be suppressed. As has been previously expressed, appropriate excitation in combination with the prevention of reflex-emergence by the clinician or client is the chief means of eventually inhibiting infantile oral activity. For example: (1) if the lower lip depresses and the jaw deviates when the angle of the mouth is stimulated (rooting reflex), the clinician should apply the appropriate stimulus and physically prevent the response from taking place; (2) if the mouth opens in response to a visual stimulus, the clinician should provide the adequate stimulus and hold the mouth closed. Whenever possible, the client himself should carry over the therapy. Two or three periods daily of such attempts at reflex-weakening is desirable.

Vegetative and Speech Breathing

Because of the frequency of primary and secondary respiratory problems in cerebral palsy and their possible effect on speech processes, it would be well for the clinician to be concerned with ensuring that each child realizes his maximum potential with respect to vegetative and speech breathing.

Clinically, improved vegetative breathing has been facilitated by the following procedures: (1) placing the individual in a supine posture, flexing the legs and pressing them toward the axillae thereby stretching the diaphragm, and then quickly returning the legs (a rhythm similar to normal vegetative breathing should be imposed); (2) occluding a single nostril with the mouth closed, thereby causing increased activity of the respiratory mechanism; (3) simulating some of the movements of the yawning reflex ("butterfly" technique) by placing the hands behind the head and initiating a head and thoracic cage dorsiflexion elbow abduction movement pattern, followed by a head and thoracic cage ventroflexion elbow adduction movement pattern (head and adducted elbows come between abducted knees); (4) fanning of the air in front of the nostrils, thereby exciting deeper inspiratory movements. In acquired cases, the above breathing procedures may also be used to good advantage.

Speech breathing activity may be facilitated by: (1) ensuring primarily an oral rather than a nasal inspiration (normal vegetative method) of air prior to voicing by occluding the nostrils before requesting the child to use his voice; (2) having the clinician, during the application of breathing techniques, stimulate so as to lengthen the expiratory phase as compared to the inspiratory phase; (3) physically resisting with the hands the beginning of an inspiratory phase for a brief period, thus causing a deeper and quicker inspiratory phase followed by a longer expiratory phase; (4) having the child hold his breath for varying periods of time to ensure a rapid and deep inspiratory phase followed by a slow and extended expiratory phase.

Vegetative and speech breathing activities should be begun as soon as respiratory problems are suspected and each activity may be done two or three times a day for five to ten minutes each time.

Obviously, it is during the periods when speech breathing activity is being stimulated that voicing should be encouraged. The clinician should utter various vowels during the expiratory phase while encouraging the child to do the same. It is hoped that this procedure should produce more spontaneous voicing on the child's part and also contribute to improving the quality and volume of his voicing as well as his ability to sustain tone for progressively longer periods of time.

Laryngeal diadochocinetic work or increasing the child's ability to alternately voice and cease voicing various vowels is also recommended.

A pertinent finding, with reference to improving respiratory activity in the cerebral palsied, has been reported by Hardy (1965). He states, ". . . An explanation of why vital capacity may be related to the speech problems of neuromuscularly handicapped speakers and not so related to speech proficiency in the normal speaker may be found by consideration of the added work load placed upon the respiratory system for speech production when paretic articulators are inefficient in their valving of the speech air stream."

Communication and Articulation

The final portion of this chapter will describe: (1) how to apply some of the ideas relative to the phylogenesis of speech in man in programs of neurospeech therapy; (2) the "neuro-conditioning" of the articulatory system; (3) the use of articulatory sensory feedback in therapy; (4) work in oral eupraxia; and (5) some general techniques on improving articulation through "amplifying" articulatory sensory feedback.

Stages in Speech Phylo-ontogenesis. The earliest, or body-head stage of communication, represents a stage where certain internal or external stimuli evoked in early man some type of generalized and nonspecific body-head activity in association with some form of unorganized vocalization. For example, primitive man's communication of impending attack might have included some generalized body movements, head gesturing, foot-stamping, arm swinging, and growl-like vocalization. Present-day reflections of this primitive stage of communication might be noted in the infant up to a month or two when he communicates discomfort and hunger by general, unorganized bodily and head movements plus crying and screaming. Older individuals may partially regress to this type of primitive communicative behavior when engaged in an emotional discussion or heated argument or when extremely frightened or angered.

The second stage or hands-face stage was reflected when early man, in his efforts at developing communication, reached the point where body postures became more organized and where bilateral hand gesturing and crude facial expressions in association with more organized and refined vocalizations became important in his signaling and communication attempts. The ontogenetic reflection of this stage may be noted during the second half of the infant's first year of life when he may extend both arms toward a parent and babble in his effort to communicate, "pick me up." An older speaker may exhibit a certain degree of this communicative behavior when he, for example, gestures and vocalizes in a noisy environment in order to lead a work crew or direct a man running a power shovel, and so on.

The face-hand stage describes that stage of intercommunication when early man developed unilateral and bilateral hand gesturing and an increased repertoire of facial expressions, plus still more re-fined phonatory and articulatory patterns. The ontogenetic reflection of this phylogenetic stage might be viewed at about 10 months or so when the child pulls himself up to a standing position, echoes syllable combinations, smiles, and makes unilateral hand gestures.

Finally, early man reached the mouth stage when his vocalizations became varied enough to allow for the development of an oral symbol system and when his facial expressions and hand gestures became coordinated and supportive communicative activities. This stage is usually reached by the infant some time during the second year of life.

Familiarity with the above ideas allows the clinician first, to assess his particular child's level of speech system evolution, and second, to co-ordinate his efforts and all others in the child's environment toward making sure that the child communicates as often as possible at that level (this means having individuals enter the child's communisphere often), at least, and is stimulated to reach the next higher level. Even the most involved child can communicate at the lowest of the levels described and hence should be encouraged to do so.

Articulatory System "Conditioning." It should prove of value if the clinician attempts to positively "condition" the muscle tone of the child's articulatory system by shaking the upper and lower lips; spreading the cheek on either side by lifting it away from the dental arch with the thumb; loosening the mandible by passively flexing and extending the mandible; loosening the tongue by lifting and bringing it over the lower incisors; and by velar stroking in order to effect better velar activity. As soon as possible, these conditioning activities should be performed daily by the child.

During these conditioning activities, the clinician should name the various articulators and eventually have the child identify them when each is touched or moved.

Articulatory Sensory Feedback. Irrespective of what the child's ar-ticulation proficiency may be, as long as it is less than desired, it is recommended that the clinician impose daily the following speech sound sensorimotor patterns upon the child's articulatory system: the bilabial pattern, by bringing the child's upper and lower lips into contact, holding them, and requesting the child to attempt to break the seal by blowing through the lips; the labiodental pattern, by lifting the child's upper lip with one hand, exposing the teeth and by raising his lower lip against the upper incisors and requesting the child to blow air through his teeth; the linguadental pattern, by placing and holding the child's tongue between his teeth and having him blow air through his teeth; the lingua-alveolar pattern, by placing the child's tongue tip against the alveolar ridge (here tongue depressor, fingers, and anything of assistance should be used) and having the child attempt to blow open the contact; the linguavelar pattern, by dorsiflexing the child's head, applying upward pressure on either side of his larynx, thereby raising the back of the tongue, and asking the child to "cough" through the point of contact.

Each of the above procedures should be done while the clinician produces simultaneously the appropriate syllable. The goal is to provide the child with more normal auditory and tactile-proprioceptive feedbacks during his attempts at speech articulation. These activities can be performed once or twice a day for brief periods with non-speaking and speaking children alike.

Oroeupraxia. The word eupraxia describes, in general, the proper performance of coordinated movements. Here, oral eupraxia describes well-performed and coordinated movements of the articulatory system.

Oroeupraxic work involves the production of an articulatory pattern which includes a base syllable plus a progressively "receding" or "preceding" syllable. For example, the production of the bilabial base syllable [bə] plus the labiodental syllable [və]. The child is asked or helped, depending on the particular child, to produce [bə-və, bə-və, etc.]. The actual production of the bilabial-labiodental combination is important and not the speed of its production. The sequence would then proceed to [bə-ðə], to [bə-də], to [bə-ʒə], to [bə-rə], and, finally, to [bə-gə]. Upon the completion of this series, the new base syllable would be [və] and the first combination would be [və-bə], then [və-ðə], and so on. The complete series of combinations would include bilabial, labiodental, linguadental, lingua-alveolar, linguapalatal, retroflex, lateral, and linguavelar base sounds and their various combinations. Again, depending on the child's potential, three and four syllable combinations may also be developed and used.

With time and after a degree of success with the movement patterns, the element of speed, or articulatory diadochocinesia, can be introduced into the oroeupraxic work. Again, such activities should be carried out for short periods of time each day.

Supportive of oroeupraxia and articulatory diadochocinesia goals is a recent finding by Hardy (1965). Hardy has shown that the severity of the speech problem in cerebral palsy is predicted better by rates of syllable repetition than by rates of nonspeech movements. Accordingly, Hardy believes that possibly the most effective way of promoting speech development in the young cerebral palsied is by eliciting attempts at actual speech productions as early as possible.

Amplifying Articulatory Sensory Feedback. It has been found that speech proficiency can be raised in various forms of adult and childhood dysarthria by techniques which appear to "amplify" sensory feedback and "gear down" speech rate. For example, in many cases of parkinsonian dysarthria and post-CVA dysarthria, simply asking the client to intentionally make harder contacts between his lips, his lips and teeth, and so on, may be found to make a good contribution to his speech proficiency. Similarly, over-articulation, slow motion articulation, and resisted articulation (fingers applying pressure to counter jaw and lip and other articulatory movements) have also proven to be useful techniques with different individuals.

Related to the speech goals is Jackson's statement: ". . . what on the lowest level are centres for movements of the tongue, palate, lips, etc., as concerned in eating, swallowing, etc., are in the highest centres evolved into the physical bases of words, symbols serving us during abstract reasoning" (1958, p. 91).

CONCLUSION

In conclusion, the major purpose of this book is to bring to the attention of cerebral palsy specialists the contribution that a neuroevolutional approach to therapy can make to the general as well as to the speech habilitation goals of the child with cerebral palsy.

Finally, it is hoped that the material has further clarified the neuroevolutional orientation for those specialists who have already begun to study the approach, and stimulated others who have not considered the orientation to begin exploring and applying the concepts and techniques.

REFERENCES

Brain, R. W. *Diseases of the Nervous System.* London: Oxford University Press, 1955.

Clement, Mary, and Twitchell, T. E. "Dysarthria in cerebral palsy," *J. Speech Hearing Dis.*, 24 (1959), 118–122.

Coriat, I. H. "The psychoanalytic conception of stammering," *The Nervous Child*, 2 (1943), 167–171.

Grewel, F. "Dysarthria in post-encephalitic parkinsonism," *Acta Psychiatrica et Neurologica*, 32 (1957), 440–449.

Hardy, J. C. "Research in Speech Problems Associated with Cerebral Palsy and Implications for the Young Cerebral Palsied" in W. T. Daley

(Ed.), *Speech and Language Therapy with the Cerebral Palsied Child.* Washington, D.C.: The Catholic University of America Press, 1965.

Head, H. "Hughlings Jackson on aphasia and kindred affections of speech," *Brain*, 38 (1915), 1–190.

Jackson, J. H. "Evolution and Dissolution of the Nervous System" in James Taylor (Ed.), *Selected Writings of John Hughlings Jackson.* Vol. 2. New York: Basic Books, Inc., 1958.

Mysak, E. D. "Significance of neurophysiological orientation to cerebral palsy habilitation," *J. Speech Hearing Dis.*, 24 (1959), 221–230.

Mysak, E. D., Pilot study films of a neurophysiological approach to cerebral palsy habilitation. Film released by the Newington Hospital for Crippled Children, Newington, Conn., June, 1960.

Mysak, E. D., Pilot study films of a neurophysiological approach to cerebral palsy habilitation: Part II. Film released by the Newington Hospital for Crippled Children, Newington, Conn., November, 1962.

Schneider, D. E. "The cortical syndromes of echolalia, echopraxia, grasping and sucking. Their significance in the disorganization of the personality," *J. New. Ment. Dis.*, 88 (1938), 18–35 and 200–216.

Sheppard, Justine J. "Cranio-oropharyngeal motor patterns in dysarthria associated with cerebral palsy," *J. Speech Hearing Res.*, 7 (1964), 373–380.

Swinyard, C. A. "Developmental aspects of neurological structure relevant to cerebral palsy," *Develop. Med. Child Neurol.*, 9 (1967), 216–221.

Ward, Marion M., Malone, Sister Henen D., Jann, Gladys R., and Jann, H. W. "Articulation variations associated with visceral swallowing and malocclusion," *J. Speech Hearing Dis.*, 26 (1961), 334–341.

Witkop, C. J., and Henry, Frances V. "Sjögren-Larsson syndrome and histidinemia: hereditary biochemical diseases with defects of speech and oral functions," *J. Speech Hearing Dis.*, 28 (1963), 109–123.

* Neuroevolution and Motor Activity

AGE	GENERAL REFLEXES AND REACTIONS	GENERAL MOTOR	AUTOMATIC HAND MOVEMENTS	INTENTIONAL HAND MOVEMENTS	ORAL REFLEXES	SPEECH
1–4 weeks	Neck Right.: present Asymm. T.N.: varies Moro: strong Upper Limb movement: present Primary infantile walking: present Primary infantile sitting: with head-leg Placing response of lower limb: present Spontaneous infantile crawling: present	Head erect:	Grasp reflex; Hand to mouth: 1 month		Rooting, lip, biting, suckling, swallowing, regurgitation: at birth	Reflexive vocalization: 0–1 month
2 months	Laby. R. on head: present Neck Right.: present Moro: present	Prone: 1–3 months	Ulnar fingers strong; grasp in pronation: 2 months		Smiling in response to maternal voice 4–6 weeks	
3 months	Primary infantile sitting: more normal position		Pulls; hands loose: 3 months Placing Response of upper limb			Babbling: 1–6 months
4–6 months	Laby. R. on head: gains Moro: diminishing Landau: commences Protect. ext. of arms: strong Arm Walking-developing Equilibrium Reaction in prone: present	Supine: 4–6 months	Clutching (body hair, dress): 4 months Scratches, rakes (ulnar): 5 months	Reaches unilaterally: 6 months	Mouth-opening to visual stimuli; laughter reflex; biting and suckling can be inhibited: 4 months	Lalling: 6–10 months

Age	General Reflexes and Reactions	General Motor	Automatic Hand Movements	Intentional Hand Movements	Oral Reflexes	Speech
7–12 months	Asymm. T.N.: present in few Landau: more frequent Body R. on body: est. in some Protect. ext. of arms: present Precipitation Reflex: present Definitive infantile walking: present Equilibrium reactions in supine and quadruped: present	Crawling: 7–8 months Sitting: 8–10 months	Slaps, scratches, rakes (whole): 7 months Radial raking; scissor grasp: 8 months Hitting; pushing; pincer grasp; waves; shakes; clasps; pokes: 10 months	Grasps string: 7 months Secures pellet (whole hand): 8 months Secures pellet (scissor grasp): 9 months Scribbles (imitation): 12 months	Chewing begins: 7 months	Echolalia: 10–12 months
12–14 months	Asymm. T.N.: disappears Landau: present in 12 of 13 Neck R.: doubtful in some Protect. ext. of arms: present Body R. on Body: change to transitional form Equilibrium reactions in sitting: present Equilibrium reactions in kneel-standing, simian stance, standing: present (12–18 months)	Standing: 12–13 months Walking: 12–18 months	Release: 12–18 months	Unwraps toy— 8½ x 11" Onion skin: 14 months		First true words: 12–18 months

* Data drawn from numerous sources including:
Berry, M. F. and Eisenson, J. *Speech Disorders: Principles and Practices of Therapy*. New York: Appleton-Century-Crofts, Inc., 1956.
Bobath, K. and Bobath, B. "Tonic reflexes and righting reflexes in the diagnosis and assessment of cerebral palsy," *Cerebral Palsy Rev.*, 16 (5) (1955), 4–10.
Cattell, P. *The Measurement of Intelligence of Infants and Young Children*. New York: The Psychological Corporation, 1940.
Gesell, A. L. et al. *The First Five Years of Life*. New York: Harper and Brothers, 1940.
Mysak, E. D. Dysarthria and oropharyngeal reflexology: a review," *J. Speech Hearing Dis.*, 28 (1963), 252–260.

Sample Forms

FORM 1. Neuroevolution and General Motor Development

Name_____ Age_____ Sex_____
Examiner_____ Date_____

1. *General Motor Development*
    (Place the child in the supine position and indicate that you wish him
    to achieve the highest motor level possible.)

Level   * *Rating*
Head raising in supine: 1_____ 2_____ 3_____ 4_____ 5_____
Side lying: _____ _____ _____ _____ _____
Head raising in prone: _____ _____ _____ _____ _____
Raises body on forearms: _____ _____ _____ _____ _____
Heel sits: _____ _____ _____ _____ _____
Assumes quadrupedal
    position: _____ _____ _____ _____ _____
Crawls: _____ _____ _____ _____ _____
Kneel-stands: _____ _____ _____ _____ _____
Kneel-walks: _____ _____ _____ _____ _____
Assumes "simian"
    position: _____ _____ _____ _____ _____
"Simian" walks: _____ _____ _____ _____ _____
Stands: _____ _____ _____ _____ _____
Walks: _____ _____ _____ _____ _____

2. *Positive Symptoms*
    (Examine child on mat.)

_____

* The ratings are defined as follows:
1. Normal
2. Mild degree of difficulty
3. Moderate degree of difficulty
4. Extreme degree of difficulty
5. No performance

Level   °° *Rating*

a. Spinal Reflexes
   flexor withdrawal: 1_____ 2_____ 3_____ 4_____ 5_____
   extensor thrust: _____ _____ _____ _____ _____
   crossed extension
      reflex: _____ _____ _____ _____ _____

b. Brain Stem Reflexes
   asymmetrical tonic
      neck: _____ _____ _____ _____ _____
   symmetrical tonic
      neck: _____ _____ _____ _____ _____
   tonic labyrinthine: _____ _____ _____ _____ _____
   positive supporting
      reaction: _____ _____ _____ _____ _____
   associated reactions: _____ _____ _____ _____ _____

c. Movement Reactions
   Moro reflex: _____ _____ _____ _____ _____
   Landau reflex: _____ _____ _____ _____ _____

3. *Righting and Equilibrium Reactions*

a. Righting Reactions (indicate highest motor level achieved via use of righting reactions, e.g., sitting, quadrupedal)

   _____

b. Equilibrium Reactions (indicate highest level of activity, e.g., in prone, sitting, quadrupedal)

   _____

4. *Evaluation*
   (Indicate level of nervous system arrestment, retardation, dissolution, e.g., Cerebral Palsy: nervous system arrestment-spinal plus brain stem level; muscle tone-moderate; motor level-supine.)

   _____
   _____

_____

°° The ratings are defined as follows:
1. Adequate stimulus evokes clear reflex or reaction, posture, or movement
2. Adequate stimulus evokes appropriate muscle tone but possibly no clear reflex, reaction, posture, or movement
3. Special stimulation such as resistance or repeated stimuli evokes reflex, reaction or appropriate tone
4. Reflex or reaction noted during performance of certain volitional acts only
5. No trace of reflex or reaction

5. *Recommendations*
   (Indicate type of treatment approach to follow, i.e., Type I, II, or III; which positive symptoms are to be concentrated on; which righting and equilibrium reactions are to be stimulated first, etc.)

   _____
   _____
   _____

FORM 2. Neuroevolution and Speech System Development

Name_____ Age_____ Sex_____
Examiner_____ Date_____

1. *Respiratory System*

a. depth of inhalation: normal_____ shallow_____
b. movements: normal_____ oppositional_____ jerky_____
c. predominant type of breathing: abdominal (diaphragmatic)_____
                                   thoracic_____
d. breaths per minute (bpm):_____

2. *Speech System Differentiation*

a. thorax from rest of body: none_____ partial_____ complete_____
b. head and neck from thorax: _____   _____   _____
c. articulators from head
     and neck: _____   _____   _____
d. articulators from each
     other: _____   _____   _____

3. *Oral Reflexology*

                                              ° *Rating*
a. palmar-mandibular
     reflex: 1_____ 2_____ 3_____ 4_____ 5_____
b. rooting reflex: _____   _____   _____   _____   _____
c. mouth opening: _____   _____   _____   _____   _____
d. lip reflex: _____   _____   _____   _____   _____
e. biting reflex: _____   _____   _____   _____   _____
f. suckling reflex: _____   _____   _____   _____   _____
g. chewing reflex: _____   _____   _____   _____   _____

4. *Negative Symptoms*
   (These reflexes are normally present throughout life and their involvement may contribute to drooling and nasality.)

° The ratings are equivalent to those used in Form 1, section 2.

a. Reflexes
   swallowing reflex: normal_____ reduced_____ strong_____
   pharyngeal reflex: _____ _____ _____
   palatal reflex: _____ _____ _____

b. Articulatory movements
   (Request child to make desired articulatory movement in syllable or
   in nonspeech form.)

1. bilabial: absent_____ incipient_____ present_____
2. labiodental: _____ _____ _____
3. linguadental: _____ _____ _____
4. lingua-alveolar: _____ _____ _____
5. linguavelar: _____ _____ _____
6. velar: _____ _____ _____

5. *Evaluation*
   (Indicate level of speech system evolution, e.g., Speech: infantile
   respiratory cycles; lack of differentiation of head and neck from thorax;
   presence of infantile oral reflex feeding complex; muscle tone-high.)

   _____
   _____

6. *Recommendations*
   (Indicate desired respiratory system approach, speech system differentiation goals, oral reflex adaptation goals, etc.)

   _____
   _____
   _____

FORM 3. Neuroevolution and Head-Arm-Hand Development

Name_____ Age_____ Sex_____
Examiner_____ Date_____

1. *Head-Arm-Hand Differentiation*

a. head and dominant arm
   from rest of body: none_____ partial_____ complete_____
b. arm from the head: _____ _____ _____
c. upper arm from the
   forearm: _____ _____ _____
d. wrist from the forearm: _____ _____ _____
e. fingers from wrist: _____ _____ _____

2. *Automatic Hand Movements*

a. *Reflexes*   * *Rating*
grasp reflex: 1_____ 2_____ 3_____ 4_____ 5_____
avoiding response: _____ _____ _____ _____ _____

b. *Basic Movements*
pulling: absent_____ incipient_____ present_____
clutching: _____   _____   _____
scratching: _____   _____   _____
raking: _____   _____   _____
slapping: _____   _____   _____
scissor grasp: _____   _____   _____
hitting: _____   _____   _____
pushing: _____   _____   _____
waving: _____   _____   _____
shaking: _____   _____   _____
pincer grasp: _____   _____   _____

3. *Evaluation*
    (Indicate level of head-arm-hand evolution, etc.)
    _____
    _____
    _____

4. *Recommendations*
    (Indicate goals for head-arm-hand differentiation, inhibition of infantile
    hand reflex, stimulation of desired automatic hand movements, etc.)
    _____
    _____
    _____

_____

    * The ratings are equivalent to those used in Form 1, section 2.

Index

111